BEAUTIFEYE

State-of-the-Art Methods to Enhance &
Rejuvenate the Eyes, Brows & Face

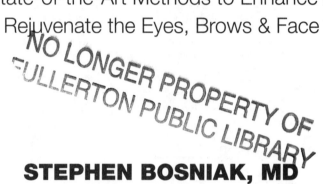
STEPHEN BOSNIAK, MD
MARIAN CANTISANO-ZILKHA, MD

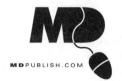

MDPUBLISH.COM

ISBN-13: 978-0-9748997-5-6
ISBN-10: 0-9748997-5-5

Printed in the United States of America.

Cover design by Nicole Sabatino
Drawings by Terri Amig
Book design by StarGraphics Studio

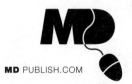

MD PUBLISH.COM   350 Fifth Avenue, Suite 7619 | New York, New York 10118

About the Authors

STEPHEN BOSNIAK, MD

Stephen Bosniak, MD is a board certified eye surgeon and cosmetic surgeon. He received his B.A from the University of Pennsylvania and his M.D. from Georgetown University. Following medical school, Dr. Bosniak completed his internship and ophthalmology residency at Washington Hospital Center in Washington, D.C. Dr. Bosniak performed a fellowship in ophthalmic plastic and reconstructive surgery at the Manhattan Eye, Ear and Throat Hospital where he is an attending surgeon.

In 1985 he edited the first book ever written on Botox®. He also has written over 150 scientific articles and has edited the nine volume series, *Advances in Ophthalmic Plastic and Reconstructive Surgery*, as well as the textbook, *Principles and Practice of Ophthalmic Plastic Surgery*, and *The Video Atlas of Cosmetic Blepharoplasty* volumes One and Two. He has written three books with Dr. Zilkha, including *Cosmetic Blepharoplasty*, *Cosmetic Blepharoplasty and Facial Rejuvenation*, and *Minimally Invasive Techniques of Oculo-Facial Rejuvenation*. He has chaired the First through the Fifth Cosmetic Eyelid Rejuvenation Symposia. He is a member of the American Society of Ophthalmic Plastic and Reconstructive Surgeons and is a member of the board of directors of the International Society of Cosmetic Laser Surgeons. In 2002 Dr. Bosniak received the prestigious Senior Achievement Award from the American Academy of Ophthalmology. He has a private practice in New York, New York.

MARIAN CANTISANO-ZILKHA, M.D.

Dr. Marian Cantisano-Zilkha, MD was trained as an eye surgeon in Rio de Janeiro, Brazil. She has been chief of the department of ophthalmology at the Central Navy Hospital in Rio. As founder and president of Total Rejuvenation Systems, she has researched and developed effective therapies that enhance and prolong the effects of surgical and non-surgical procedures. She has revolutionized non-traumatic micropigmentation (semi-permanent make-up) techniques that dramatize the final results of laser blepharoplasty. She is the co-author with Dr. Bosniak of *Cosmetic Blepharoplasty and Facial Rejuvenation, Minimally Invasive Techniques of Oculo-Facial Rejuvenation*, and the *Second Video Atlas of Cosmetic Blepharoplasty*. She has co-chaired the Fourth and Fifth Cosmetic Eyelid Rejuvenation Symposia and has lectured extensively in Europe and South America. She is a member of the International Society of Cosmetic Laser Surgeons and the American Society for Laser Medicine and Surgery. Dr. Zilkha is the director of oculoplastic surgery at The Ipanema Center for Cosmetic and Reconstructive Eyelid Surgery in Rio de Janeiro, Brazil, where she has developed techniques for products before they were available in the United States. She has her private practice in Rio.

BOSNIAK+ZILKHA

Bosniak+Zilkha have performed surgical demonstrations for doctors on five continents to instruct them on cosmetic and reconstructive eyelid surgical techniques as well as non-invasive facial rejuvenation procedures. They are members of the Botox® National Teaching Network. Their last textbook *Non-Invasive Techniques of Oculo-Facial Rejuvenation* (Thieme Publishers, New York) was released in May 2005 and is being translated into Portuguese. It is available directly from the publisher (**www.Thieme.com** in the ophthalmology section). A list of their published textbooks is available in the reference section at the back of this book. For the complete list of their scientific publications go to **www.eye-lift.com**, meet the doctors, curriculum vitae.

TEXTBOOKS WRITTEN BY STEPHEN BOSNIAK & MARIAN CANTISANO-ZILKHA, M.D.

Bosniak, Stephen L., Marian Cantisano-Zilkha. *Minimally Invasive Techniques of Oculo-Facial Rejuvenation*, Thieme Medical Publishers, Inc., 2005.

Bosniak, Stephen L., Marian Cantisano-Zilkha. *Blefaroplastia Cosmetica Y Rejuvenecimiento Facial*—Segundo Edicion Amolca, Madrid, Spain, 2004.

Bosniak, Stephen L., Marian Cantisano-Zilkha. *Cosmetic Blepharoplasty & Facial Rejuvenation*, Lippincott-Raven: Philadelphia, 1999.

Bosniak, Stephen L., Cantisano-Zilkha, Marian. *Video Atlas of Cosmetic Blepharoplasty, Vol. 2, Essentials of Contemporary Surgical Approaches*, Medical Video Productions: St. Louis, Mo., 1996.

Bosniak, Stephen L. *The Principles & Practice of Ophthalmic Plastic & Reconstructive Surgery, Vol. 1 & 2*, WB Saunders: Philadelphia, 1995.

Bosniak, Stephen L. *Video Atlas of Cosmetic Blepharoplasty*. St. Louis: Medical Video Productions, 1992.

Bosniak, Stephen and Byron C. Smith. *Advances in Ophthalmic, Plastic, and Reconstructive Surgery:The Orbital Trauma Part 2., Vol 9*, New York: Pergamon Press, 1990.

Bosniak, Stephen L. *Cosmetic Blepharoplasty*. Raven Press, 1990.

Bosniak, Stephen and Byron C. Smith. *Advances in Ophthalmic, Plastic, and Reconstructive Surgery:The Orbital Trauma Part 1., Vol 8*, New York: Pergamon Press, 1989.

Bosniak, Stephen, Smith, Byron. *Advances in Ophthalmic Plastic and Reconstructive Surgery—Complex Socket Deformities, Vol. 7*, New York: Pergamon Press, 1988.

Bosniak, Stephen L., Smith, Byron. *Advances in Ophthalmic Plastic and Reconstructive Surgery -The Anophthalmic Socket., Vol. 6*, New York: Pergamon Press, 1987.

Bosniak, Stephen L., Smith, Byron. *Advances in Ophthalmic Plastic and Reconstructive Surgery: History and Tradition, Vol. 5*, New York: Pergamon Press, 1986.

Bosniak, Stephen L., Smith, Byron. *Advances in Ophthalmic Plastic and Reconstructive Surgery:Blepharospasm, Vol. 4*, New York: Pergamon Press, 1985.

Bosniak, Stephen L., Smith, Byron. A*dvances in Ophthalmic, Plastic, and Reconstructive Surgery:The Lacrimal System, Vol. 3*, New York: Pergamon Press, 1984.

Bosniak, Stephen L., Smith, Byron. *Advances in Ophthalmic Plastic and Reconstructive Surgery:The Aging Face, Vol. 2*, New York: Pergamon Press, 1983.

Bosniak, Stephen L., Smith, Byron. *Advances in Ophthalmic Plastic and Reconstructive Surgery—Ptosis, Vol One*, New York: Pergamon Press, 1982.

Acknowledgments

To our North American and Brazilian staff who create an efficient and comforting ambience for our patients— Joan Sabatino, Danielle Braz, Pamela Petti, Ana Lucia Caldas, Dr. Ana Farinha, Marie Theresa Fatorelli, Margarida Guimaraes, Cristina Guidoni, Alessandra Sales de Barros, Samantha Bittencourt Suprani, the late beloved Dr. Afonso Fatorelli, Dr. Miguel Angelo Padilha, Dr. Renato Ambrosio Jr., and Dr. Israel Rozemberg. To Audrey Kitagawa for editorial insights. To Julie Fanelli, Cee Cee Yarabinee, and Patricia Doyle of Esthetica Spa. To Denice Monaco. And to our fellows, Dr. Ioannis Glavas, Dr. Lisa Zidinak, Dr. Baljeet Purewal, Dr. Rachel Ellis, and Dr. Susan Burekhovich.

*To our patients who inspire us
to always strive for the very best in
professional care and service.*

Contents

Foreword

Stephen Bosniak and Marian Cantisano-Zilkha have introduced what is arguably one of the most comprehensive books on facial and eye rejuvenation therapies, including the latest non-surgical procedures, anti-oxidant protocols and laser treatments.

The difference between how the surgery was performed twenty years ago as compared with today, is like comparing the covered wagon to an SUV. Drs. Bosniak and Cantisano-Zilkha have been leaders and innovators in the field, allowing their patients to feel comfortable that their procedures will be successful. These techniques are outlined in this seminal book.

The BOSNIAK+ZILKHA team was created in 1995 after the First Brazilian Congress on Ophthalmic Plastic and Reconstructive Surgery. Since then, Drs. Bosniak and Zilkha have written two textbooks and dozens of scientific articles, compiled a video atlas, and lectured and performed surgical demonstrations on five continents.

Dr. Bosniak's scholarship is well documented, as he wrote the first book on Botox® in 1985. In addition, he has written over one hundred scientific articles and has edited the nine volume series *Advances in Ophthalmic Plastic & Reconstructive Surgery*. He has authored the textbooks *Cosmetic Blepharoplasty, Principles & Practice of Ophthalmic Plastic & Reconstructive Surgery* and *The Video Atlas of Cosmetic Blepharoplasty, Volume One*.

Dr. Zilkha maintains a prestigious cosmetic and reconstructive ophthalmic plastic surgical practice in Rio de Janeiro, Brazil. She directed the first major clinical study using Restylane® for facial rejuvenation in her clinic there.

As if this were not impressive enough, together, Drs. Bosniak and Zilkha have written *Cosmetic Blepharoplasty and Facial Rejuvenation*, and *Non Invasive Techniques of*

Facial Rejuvenation. They have authored *The Video Atlas of Cosmetic Blepharoplasty, Volume Two.* They have also chaired the First through Fifth Cosmetic Eyelid Rejuvenation Symposia and have been actively involved in the education of aestheticians.

Drs. Bosniak and Zilkha are members of the International Society of Cosmetic Laser Surgeons, the American Society for Laser Medicine and Surgery and the advisory board of the Asia-Pacific Society of Ophthalmic Plastic and Reconstructive Surgeons. Dr. Bosniak has been widely recognized for his *nonpareil work*, having received the prestigious Senior Achievement Award from the American Academy of Ophthalmology in 2004 and having been selected to the board of directors of the International Society of Cosmetic Laser Surgeons.

Enjoy this book. It is a treasure.

—Gary Null

Gary Null is a nationally syndicated talk show host and producer of PBS *specials, a consumer advocate, investigative reporter,* New York Times *best-selling author and an award-winning documentary filmmaker.*

Preface

WHY WE WROTE THIS BOOK

What prompted us to write this book was our desire to inform you—the public—by providing a comprehensive view of the current non-invasive facial cosmetic treatments available. Having proper information will help you to make better and appropriate choices in your decision to undertake steps to improve your appearance. Feeling satisfied with your appearance can enhance self esteem, motivate you to take better care of yourself, and be the impetus to improve the overall quality of your life. Surgery is no longer the only path to helping you recapture and retain that fresh, vibrant look. These non-surgical treatments which we describe in this book can forestall, and in some cases, eliminate entirely, the need for surgery. Our laser surgical techniques have minimized recovery time and complications, but increasingly, people seek a less intimidating approach as a first step to avoid the problems and risks which surgery can pose. We lead busy lives and are looking for ways in which we can receive the benefits of treatment which improve our appearance with minimal or no downtime.

—Stephen Bosniak, MD
—Marian Cantisano-Zilkha, MD
www.eye-lift.com
www.beautifeye.com

Introduction

"Beauty is truth, truth beauty,—that is all ye know on earth, and all ye need to know."—John Keats

"Beauty is a greater recommendation than any letter of introduction."—Aristotle

What is the first thing you notice about a person? It is almost always their eyes. The eyes establish immediate contact when people interact.

The subtle contours of the eyelid area significantly contribute to the overall appearance of the face. If the eyelids are drooping or bulging, the face projects a look of fatigue and lack of vigor despite adequate rest and good health. If the eyes look bright and alert, the effect of a sagging jaw line or neck may seem less important. The position of the eyebrows and eyelids can convey many emotions, from anger to sadness, even when a person is experiencing no such emotion.

The increasingly recognized field of ophthalmic plastic and reconstructive surgery is a highly specialized area of ophthalmology that deals with cosmetic enhancements of the eyelid area, as well as the management of deformities of the eyelids, eyebrows, upper face, the tear drainage system, and the orbital bones that surround the eye. Surgery around the eyes can affect the function as well as the appearance of the eyes. As oculoplastic surgeons, we are specially trained to perform this delicate surgery while improving eyelid function, enhancing eyelid appearance and protecting the integrity of the eye itself. The delicate, rapid movements of the eyelids must be kept in perfect balance and maintain perfect contact with the eye itself.

Our evolution into eyelid and facial rejuvenation was actually inspired by our patients. We noticed that many of the patients who were referred to us for correction of eyelid problem from accidents, tumors, or complications of surgery performed by other physicians did not know that there were doctors who specialized in eyelid surgery. Many of these patients also had complaints about their aging eyelids.

> • *I spent a lot of time in the sun, and now I have crow's feet around my eyes.*
>
> • *I am young but because I have bags under my eyes, my co-workers think I am not getting enough sleep or I am always tired.*
>
> • *When I wear eye shadow, it smudges and does not stay on.*
>
> • *My body is in good shape, but my eyes make me look tired and older than I really am.*
>
> • *I have tried many eye creams with no results.*
>
> • *My eyes have always been my best feature. As I have gotten older, they seem to be getting smaller.*

Because there are two of us—a man and a woman—we can give you our insights from two different perspectives. After working together for so many years, each of us has learned to understand and appreciate the other's point of view.

There are small details on a woman's face that men cannot see because testosterone affects their retinas.

In the film, "What Women Want," (2000), a man finds himself getting an unexpected crash course in the psychology of contemporary women. Nick Marshall (Mel Gibson) is an advertising executive who thinks of himself as a ladies' man, although he has little understanding of women beyond figuring out how to seduce them. After Nick is shocked in an electrical accident in his bathroom, he discovers that he can hear what women are thinking. This is a revelation to him.

Women are more critical than men, and they can be hyper- critical of themselves and of other women. Sometimes a small wrinkle or depression that men barely notice may disturb a woman tremendously when she looks in the mirror. Men look at women entirely differently. They respond to the overall image of women, often overlooking seemingly minute details. If a male physician dismisses these imperfections that he thinks are insignificant, he may alienate his patient. Conversely, men will analyze a problem differently than women and often create a different solution. It is clear that having both perspectives is a great advantage.

We are bombarded daily with information about all the new and improved surgical and non-surgical techniques now available. They are written up in beauty magazines and discussed on TV talk shows. How would you know which procedures work and which are just hype? How would you know which procedures are appropriate for you? In this book we will share our preferences with you, based upon our years of experience, and our commitment to providing our patients with the safest, maximally effective, and minimally invasive techniques available.

We perceive the doctor-patient relationship, as one built upon the clear understanding of your realistic expectations and designing a treatment program that will be the safest and best for you in the long run. So for example, if we can improve the quality, texture, and resilience of your skin, this may not only postpone the need for surgery, but may actually improve the surgical result when we do perform the procedure at some time in the future.

THE BRAZILIAN CONNECTION

In Rio de Janeiro, where the well-rounded rock formations that surround the city suggest the sensuous bodies of the Brazilian women and the sun beats down intensely all year long, the beach is the center of business meetings and social life. The result is SUN DAMAGE. Not everyone in Brazil is dark-skinned. The ethnic diversity in Brazil is extreme—from the strong African influence in Bahia to the German and Italian communities in Santa Catarina. This has given us extensive experience in countering the effects of the sun in all skin types.

CORRECT, PROTECT, RENEW™

New insights into the facial aging process and the discovery of advanced technology have led us to develop an innovative approach to non-invasive rejuvenation of the upper face —"CORRECT, PROTECT, RENEW"™. Improvements in terms of simplicity, lack of downtime, comfort, efficiency, and safety have greatly increased our patients' acceptance and desire for these procedures.

We want this book to be your guide to "correct, protect, renew"™ your eyes, brows, and face. And so we have provided a series of flow charts and short cuts:

• **CORRECT**—quick reference maps for showing you the best non-invasive techniques for correcting the effects of sun damage and aging.

• **PROTECT**—easy to follow diagrams to help you care for your eyes and face.

• **RENEW**—flow charts to guide you through your choices of minimally invasive procedures.

Each chapter will also include very detailed descriptions of all of the non-surgical and surgical procedures if you care to delve into any of the topics in greater depth. Please enjoy this book, read it, study it, take it with you to your doctors' offices. You can contact us through the websites below.

—Stephen Bosniak, MD
—Marian Cantisano-Zilkha, MD
www.eye-lift.com
www.beautifeye.com

CHAPTER 1

Your Eyes
Are Your
Calling Card

Our philosophy is to respect every patient as an individual, entitled to the best professional service possible, through the safest, least invasive, and most advanced medical techniques available.

How do you know when you are ready for intervention?

The goal of an eyelift is to improve the appearance and function of your eyelids by using the least detectable method that produces the most natural-looking results.

You should be motivated to do something about your eyes when you see something that bothers you—new wrinkles, folds, creases, sagging, or heavy bags. In more severe cases you may actually have physical complaints; a heavy upper lid may block out some of your peripheral vision, or push your eyelashes against your eye causing the impulse to brush something away from your eye. Heavy upper lids can give you a frontal headache at the end of the day because the frontalis muscle in the forehead has been working so hard to keep the eyebrows and eyelids elevated and out of your field of vision. These bothersome discoveries are not only related to age, but may be familial traits or tendencies.

The goal of an eyelift is to improve the appearance and function of your eyelids in a natural, undetectable way. That is why old photographs are so important. Everyone's eyelids are structurally different. Everyone's fold, crease, and relationship to the eyebrow and angle of the outside corner (lateral canthus) is different. No two eyelifts are exactly alike. Many patients who have come to us after a facelift look beautiful. Their job was technically perfect, but we did not recognize them. If someone sees you and says, "*Nice eye job*," it is not.

Our overriding goal is to make you look better, not make you look like someone else.

It is important for your doctor to embrace a variety of therapies, utilizing surgical options as well as injectable treatments (botulinum toxin, fillers, mesotherapy), lasers and light sources, and radio-frequency energy. A doctor who is well versed in a variety of therapies has a larger capacity to meet your needs with methods appropriate for you.

What do the eyelids do?

The eyelids protect the eye from injury. They regulate the light that reaches the eye. The eyelids distribute the protective and optically important tear film over the cornea during blinking, and they regulate tear out flow by their pumping action. If your eyelid muscles are too loose, your eyes will tear because your eyelid muscles are not pushing the tears into the tear drains.

The eyelids are obviously much more complex than you may think they are. There are two muscles in each eyelid that open the eyelid and a muscle that encircles your eyelids to close them. Understanding the structure of the area around the eyes will reveal many clues as to the changes that appear with aging.

THE ORBIT

The orbital bones around the eye form a protective cone shaped cave. These orbital bones help define the level and contour of your eyebrows and cheek bones.

What do the eyebrows do?

The eyebrows have an important cosmetic function; they are a defining facial feature, creating a facial balance and a frame for the eyes. The eyebrows also have a protective function since the hairs keep liquids from dripping into the eyes and foreign bodies away from the eyes.

What is a glabella?

The glabella is the anatomic area between the eyebrows.

Several muscles in this area are responsible for facial expressions, for example, the expression of concern or frowning, referred to as "Your 11".

The upper eyelid extends up to the eyebrow, which separates it from the forehead. The level and contour of the eyebrows will affect the upper eyelid folds. If the eyebrow droops (eyebrow ptosis) the upper eyelid fold will be heavy.

You will not receive demerits if you cannot name the brow depressors. But you should know that there are muscles that pull your brows down and muscles that lift your brows up. You should know that we can change the shape and levels of your eyebrows by readjusting the balance of these muscles with Botox®, Thermage®, fillers, lasers, and surgery.

THE BROW MUSCLES	
MUSCLE	**WHAT IT DOES**
CORRUGATOR	A brow depressor, just above the brow that creates vertical frown lines ("Your 11")
PROCERUS	A brow depressor; creates horizontal lines at the base of the nose
FRONTALIS	A brow elevator; muscle of entire forehead that elevates brows, creates horizontal furrows; when your upper eyelids are heavy or droop, the frontalis automatically elevates the brows and pulls the drooping eyelid out of the visual axis—like raising a window shade—to improve peripheral vision.
ORBICULARIS	Really an eyelid muscle, but also pulls the eyebrow down—a brow depressor; also creates "crows feet"

MIDFACE

The tissues of the midface begin at the level of the cheek bone below the eyelid, and are not formally part of the eyelid. However, the lower eyelid and cheek combine to form a single functional unit. Of course there is fatty tissue in the lower eyelid that can create bags, but sometimes there is also fat over the cheekbone that can create a "bag on a bag"—a cheek bag. This will not be corrected with a standard eyelift, but it can be improved with laser resurfacing or Thermage® to tighten the tissue.

The midface also has a support function for the lower lid. Looseness of the midfacial muscles and skin can also contribute to lower eyelid laxity.

There are numerous muscles of the midface that are responsible for facial expression and animation. Sometimes these muscles can create lower lid wrinkles and folds.

WHAT ARE MY CHOICES?
"CORRECT, PROTECT, RENEW"™

Lifts lift the skin and tissues, fillers fill up creases, lasers and peels resurface, and botulinum toxin softens muscle activity. Each method has its place, and one does not always do the job of the other. They all work together.

A combination of treatments is done in phases. Treatment for improving skin quality and texture with light and non-ablative (no downtime) laser devices, also referred to as photorejuvenation and photodynamic therapy, is best approached in a sensible, stepwise fashion. We often recommend performing procedures in a specific order. For example, we may use botulinum toxin to relax the muscles and then treat the skin with chemical peels before radiofrequency therapy for skin tightening.

The real beauty of this vast array of choices is that each

category complements the other and that a combination of treatments may work better than any of them by themselves. Many of our patients, both women and men, are concentrating on minimally invasive procedures combined with good skincare to forestall the need for surgery. These treatments are considered alternatives to going under the knife, or adjuncts to cosmetic surgery that enhance and maintain the results.

You have choices. To help you understand your options each of the following chapters will describe in great detail how each of these different treatments work. These treatments will be separated into different categories: skin texture, skin pigmentation, skin wrinkling, skin looseness (laxity), skin excess, skin depressions, and skin folds. Specific areas of the face will be addressed: the eyebrows, the upper eyelids, the lower eyelids, the midface, the lower face, the jowls, and the neck.

We have provided a step by step flow chart for guiding you from one level of treatment to the next.

The eyelid flow chart (FIG 1) will take you through the process of improving eyelid texture and contour, one step at a time, from the completely non-invasive to the minimally invasive.

Your Eyes

Begin with twice a day applications of our newly developed Beautif-Eye™ cream to your upper and lower eyelid. Add in-office peels and CO2Cellulair™. These first two steps will begin to improve skin texture and pigmentation. Add Botox® treatments to further decrease, but not eliminate, dynamic expression lines. Tighten the eyelid skin with the new Thermage® eyelid hand piece. Support your brows and fill in eyelid depressions with Restylane®. Pursue further lifting and tightening with a BZ lift, then laser resurfacing, and finally a full laser-assisted eyelift with tendon tightening. At

| FIG. 1 | Eyelid Flow Chart |

GO WITH THE FLOW: A step by step flow chart for guiding you from one level of treatment to the next. What to do when you want to crank up your results a notch.

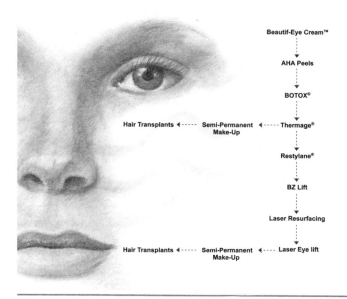

RENEW: EYE FLOW CHART (FIG 1)

There is an order of procedures that we follow, starting from the simplest to the slightly more involved. We begin with topical products that we have developed and have found to be effective, and then add from our menu of procedures, one step at a time. We advance until we have achieved a result that you are satisfied with. Semi-permanent make-up can be added at any step.

any point you may add eyebrow and eyelash rejuvenation to your wish list. Micropigmentation—semi-permanent make-up—and then even single hair transplants are techniques used to fill out your brows and lashes.

The face flow chart (**FIG 2**) will take you step by step from the non-invasive to the minimally invasive treatments to rejuvenate your face:

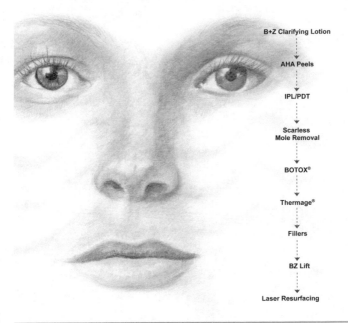

| FIG. 2 | **Face Flow Chart** |

GO WITH THE FLOW: A step by step flow chart for guiding you from one level of treatment to the next. What to do when you want to crank up your results a notch.

B+Z Clarifying Lotion
↓
AHA Peels
↓
IPL/PDT
↓
Scarless Mole Removal
↓
BOTOX®
↓
Thermage®
↓
Fillers
↓
BZ Lift
↓
Laser Resurfacing

RENEW: FACE FLOW CHART (FIG 2)

There is an order of procedures that we follow, starting from the simplest to the slightly more involved. We begin with topical products that we have developed and have found to be effective, and then add from our menu of procedures, one step at a time. We advance until we have achieved a result that you are satisfied with. Laser surgical procedures are our final step.

CORRECT (FIGURES 3, 4 & 5)

Correct the texture and tone of your eyelids with Beautif-Eye™ cream in the morning, loaded with super Brazilian rain forest moisturizers, Brazilian rain forest botanical anti-oxidants, and high-tech skin relaxers to simulate a mild Botox®-like effect. Even pigmentation with B+Z clarifying lotion, prescription

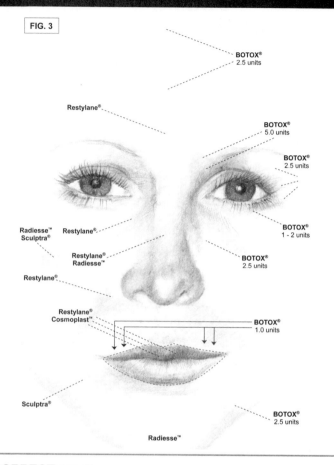

FIG. 3

BOTOX®
2.5 units

Restylane®

BOTOX®
5.0 units

BOTOX®
2.5 units

BOTOX®
1 - 2 units

Radiesse™
Sculptra®

Restylane®

Restylane®
Radiesse™

BOTOX®
2.5 units

Restylane®

Restylane®
Cosmoplast™

BOTOX®
1.0 units

Sculptra®

BOTOX®
2.5 units

Radiesse™

CORRECT (FIG 3)

We use BOTOX® to relax muscles in the face, to soften wrinkles
around your eyes, to remove "your number 11", to lift your brows,
to raise the corners of your mouth, to smoothen out your upper lip
lines, and to ease your neck bands. Because each muscle is different,
we use a different dose for each muscle.

We use different fillers for different parts of the face. For shallow
furrows between your eyebrows or in your forehead we fill with
Restylane. For deeper folds between your nose and mouth, Perlane.
For hollow cheeks, Sculptra. For augmenting your cheek bones and
chin, Radiesse. To accentuate your lip, Restylane, Cosmoplast, Juvé-
derm, Restylane Lipp, Perlane. And around your mouth, a combination of fillers.

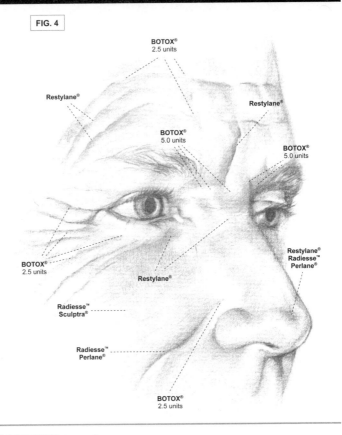

FIG. 4

BOTOX®
2.5 units

Restylane®

Restylane®

BOTOX®
5.0 units

BOTOX®
5.0 units

Restylane®
Radiesse™
Perlane®

BOTOX®
2.5 units

Restylane®

Radiesse™
Sculptra®

Radiesse™
Perlane®

BOTOX®
2.5 units

CORRECT (FIG 4)

In men, the strength of the facial muscles are greater and the depths of the folds are typically deeper. We use higher doses of Botox® and thicker fillers for our non-invasive techniques in men.

strength skin lighteners with retinols. Super charge your homecare products with in-office, no-downtime fruit acid peels and CO2Cellulair™ treatment. Relax wrinkle-causing muscles around your eyes, forehead, and brow depressors with Botox®, giving you a brow lift. The new Thermage® eyelid tip will tighten and lift your eyelid skin. Restylane® will

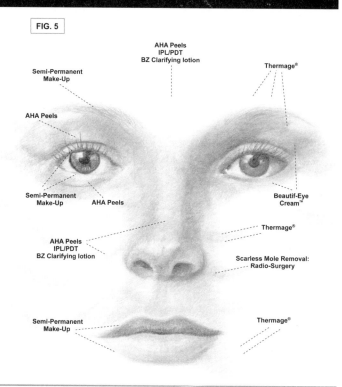

FIG. 5

AHA Peels
IPL/PDT
BZ Clarifying lotion

Thermage®

Semi-Permanent
Make-Up

AHA Peels

Semi-Permanent
Make-Up   AHA Peels

Beautif-Eye
Cream™

AHA Peels
IPL/PDT
BZ Clarifying lotion

Thermage®

Scarless Mole Removal:
Radio-Surgery

Semi-Permanent
Make-Up

Thermage®

CORRECT (FIG 5)

To complement facial filling and muscle relaxation, we improve skin texture with homecare products, peels, CO2Cellulair™, IPL, photo-dynamic therapy. We tighten and lift with Thermage and the Alma ST handpiece, and other radio frequency and infrared devices.

fill in depressions not completely corrected with Botox® and Thermage®, give additional brow support, and fill in the shadowy depressions under your eyes. Remove moles and precancerous lumps and bumps with scarless mole removal—radiosurgery. Raise the eyebrows and tighten forehead and eyelid skin with Thermage®. Combining all of these non-invasive lifting techniques with a BZ Lift—so unique that it is patent pending.

Eyes

Beautif-Eye™ cream
Make-up with sun screen

Beautif-Eye™ cream's powerful anti-oxidants will help to reverse sun damage and keep the delicate eyelid skin well hydrated. Chemical free sunscreens with physical sun blocking power will keep out UVA, UVC, and UVB rays. Standard sun screens do NOT protect against UVA and UVC.

CORRECT. **PROTECT**. RENEW.™

FIG. 6

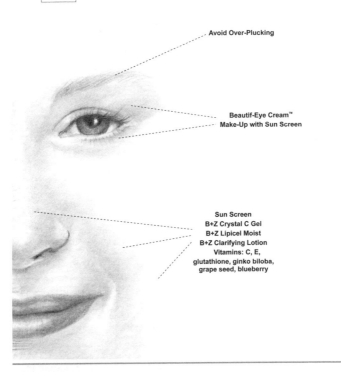

Avoid Over-Plucking

Beautif-Eye Cream™
Make-Up with Sun Screen

Sun Screen
B+Z Crystal C Gel
B+Z Lipicel Moist
B+Z Clarifying Lotion
Vitamins: C, E,
glutathione, ginko biloba,
grape seed, blueberry

PROTECT (FIG 6)

Use sunscreens daily, applying them generously and often. To protect your facial skin we recommend topical and oral anti-oxidants for extra protection.

Brows

To preserve your eyebrow hairs avoid over-plucking. Over-plucking can destroy the hair follicles. Micropigmentation—semi-permanent make-up—can often stimulate eyebrow hair growth.

The first step in protecting your face is to make the use of sun screen part of your year-round daily routine. UVB rays burn your skin when the sun is shining. But UVA and UVC rays are bombarding your skin whether the sun is out or not, even if you are inside next to a window. You must also realize that sun screens are NOT a complete sun block. They must be reapplied every two to three hours, and they must be applied thickly. A thin layer of sun screen will only give a fraction of the SPF quoted on the tube. To take care of the free radicals in your skin that get past your sun screen you need to apply topical anti-oxidants and take them internally as well. Some of the most potent—and our favorites—are: vitamins C and E, glutathione, selenium, Ginko Biloba, grape seed and blueberry extracts, taken as capsules twice daily. Our B+Z clarifying lotion will fade abnormal pigmentation caused by the sun and stimulate skin repair.

After you have followed the first steps for non-invasive CORRECTION and then followed a basic regimen for PROTECTION, the motivation to do something about these symptoms should come from you, not because someone else says that you need it. Once you are certain that you want to proceed, you should investigate all your options. Not all the options are surgical. From an ever-expanding menu of minimally invasive, non-surgical options, you can proceed to RENEW.

RENEW (FIGURE 7)

Eyes

Laser resurfacing
Laser Eye lift
Laser tendon tightening
Laser muscle repositioning
Laser fat repositioning
Semi-permanent eye-liner
Eye lash transplantation

FIG. 7 | **MINIMALLY INVASIVE PROCEDURES**

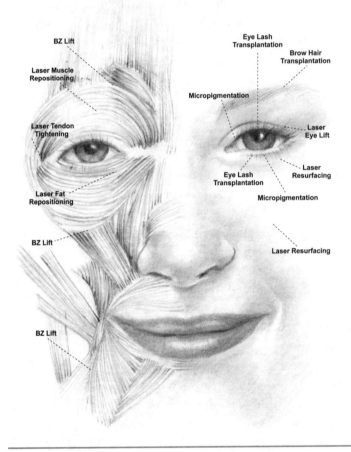

BZ Lift

Laser Muscle Repositioning

Laser Tendon Tightening

Laser Fat Repositioning

BZ Lift

BZ Lift

Eye Lash Transplantation

Brow Hair Transplantation

Micropigmentation

Laser Eye Lift

Laser Resurfacing

Eye Lash Transplantation

Micropigmentation

Laser Resurfacing

RENEW (FIG 7)

Our minimally invasive procedures with lasers and radio frequency devices can reposition lax tissues and restore the resilience to skin, muscles and supportive tendons, keeping downtime to a minimum.

So the creams, lotions, peels, and injectable therapies have improved the appearance of your eyes, but not enough. It is time to consider laser eyelid skin resurfacing and even a full laser-assisted lift. Using the laser as an incisional tool rather than a scalpel will cut your healing time in half. Tightening your supportive tendons and repositioning muscles will make your eyelids more youthful but without that overdone, deer in the headlights look. Avoiding any skin incisions in your lower eyelids will avoid any unwanted change in your eye shape. Shifting your lower lid fat pockets without removing them entirely will make your undereye area naturally smooth and not too hollowed out.

As the final touch, rejuvenating your eyebrows and eyelashes with micropigmentation and even some new hairs will frame your eyes beautifully.

Brows

BZ Lift
Semi-permanent brow make-up
Brow hair transplantation
Laser Brow Lift

Putting your eyebrows in the right position is the key to a successful eyelift. If necessary and to complement our non-invasive, no-downtime BZ lift, then our laser-assisted technique of placing internal supportive stitches from an upper eyelid crease opening will give you a refreshed look without any additional incisions in your forehead or hairline.

CHAPTER 2

The Youthful Eye, How It Ages, & What You Can Do About It

Aging around the eyelids is, to a large extent, determined by heredity. If you have saggy or baggy eyelids, your parents and siblings probably have them too.

The eye area is the first facial area to show the effects of time and lifestyle, and where fine wrinkles first appear. The eyelid skin is the thinnest in the body, and is always exposed to environmental aggressions such as wind, low temperatures, UV rays, dust, and pollution. This thin skin is subject to stress, fatigue, and thus, early signs of aging.

A well-positioned brow, a crisp upper lid fold, smooth, evenly pigmented skin, and full eyelashes are the signs of a youthful upper lid. A deep upper eyelid is not youthful and is no longer considered a good result following blepharoplasty. A youthful lower eyelid has a firm lower lid margin that fits tightly against the eye and has a sharp, acute outer angle that slants slightly upward. The skin is evenly pigmented and smooth, and there are no shadows or irregularities from bulging fat.

The Differences Between Women & Men

The level, shape and contour of the eyelids are different in women and men. The brows are generally more arched and higher in women than in men. But the ultra high, arched woman's brow of the 30's and 40's does not give a natural look is no longer acceptable. In men, there is a shorter distance between the eyebrows and eyelashes. The vertical height of their upper lids is less. The brow itself is more horizontal and lower. Some dynamic wrinkles are more acceptable for men.

EYELID SKIN

The delicate skin of the eyelids is the thinnest skin of the body, and it is easily effected by the environment.

The eyelids are delicate and complex. They have to blink hundreds of times a minute to constantly refresh the tear film and keep the corneas moist. There is an upper eyelid crease that allows the upper lid to open and close quite easily. It is also an important anatomic landmark. It is where the opening muscle of the eyelid attaches to the skin. This is where we hide our incisions when performing an upper eyelid lift or repairing a drooping upper lid. This fold becomes heavy as the skin loses its elasticity and becomes fuller when the brow droops. If too much of this skin is removed during eyelid surgery, the fold becomes too tight and the eye will not close completely.

Even though the eyelid is so thin, its structure is very complex. Seven layers of tissue make up the upper eyelid.

LOWER EYELID

Some surgeons make lower lid skin incisions just under the lower lid eyelashes, which may remain visible as a slight indentation. This technique can also result in too much white showing under the eye—lower lid retraction.

Tendons—attached to the orbital bones that surround the eye—support the lower lid, keeping it in the proper position and holding it tight against the eye.

Nervous ticks or blepharospasm are a result of uncontrolled eyelid muscle contractions, causing the eyes to close when you do not want them to. Relieving these involuntary muscle contractions was one of the first uses of botulinum toxin.

EYELID AGING CHANGES

Faces age in a predictable manner. Genetics influence how much age-related changes will affect you.

THE 30's	Thin skin of the eyelids starts to lose its elasticity and stretch. In the upper eyelids, the skin may start to hang over the

THE 30's	crease. As the collagen degrades, wrinkles and crow's feet appear in the parts of the eyelids that are most mobile. There is little excess skin in the upper lids. The earliest signs of genetic predispositions may begin to show. Fat may bulge through the lower eyelid skin. Full upper eyelids may begin to appear heavy.
THE 40's	Upper eyelid skin begins to overhang the upper eyelid crease. The skin is less elastic and fat may bulge through. Crow's feet form around the eyes; dynamic frown depressions between the eyebrows begin to show. Lower lid shadows created by bulging fat start to show. Under eye dark circles become more noticeable. Sun damage will be visible as areas of spots and patches of skin darkening, fine lines, and broken capillaries.
THE 50's	Gravitational effects become more pronounced. Drooping of the outer aspect of the eyebrows becomes evident. Further progression of genetic and environmental factors. More wrinkling and pigmentary changes. Animated facial expressions result in more wrinkling. Skin texture is not as firm, upper lid folds are not as well-defined. Shadowing and irregularities of the eyelid contours are visible. Lower eyelids do not fit as tightly against the eye. The outside (lateral canthal) angles are not as sharp.
THE 60's & BEYOND	The upper eyelid margin droops as the tendon of the eyelid lifting muscle (levator) thins, and the brow drops. Outer corners of the eyes become blunted and lose their upward slant, lower lid sagging (inferior scleral show) gives the eyes a

The Aging Lower Lid—Cheek Complex

Just as the eyebrow and upper lid are related and the brow position effects the upper eyelid fold, the lower eyelid and cheek are related. The supportive muscles and subcutaneous tissues of both are connected. Supporting loose tendons will redrape the lower eyelid tissues. Repositioning of the lower eyelid fat pockets instead of removing lower lid fat gives a better and more youthful contour. Elevating the midface can also improve lower eyelid support and contour. We avoid cutting the lower eyelid skin during any of our surgical procedures as this can pull the eyelids down. We prefer the less invasive approaches to the midface—Thermage® to tighten and lift the skin and internal stitches when necessary.

Changes also occur in the upper cheek area. In youth, the lower eyelid muscle lies flat over the cheekbone. With time, this muscle loses tone and can create a bulge. When there is an extra fold of skin, muscle, and fat on the cheek, this is called a malar festoon or a bag on a bag. The soft tissues of the cheek and midface (fat, muscles, supportive fascia) lose tone and descend, and some subcutaneous fat is also lost, exposing a small area of hollowness below the lower eyelid, accentuating lower eyelid imperfections, and allowing the edge of the orbital bone to show through the skin (a change known as skeletonization.) The combination of the downward shifting of the facial skin, muscle, and subcutaneous tissue, with the loss of fat and bone volume creates a flattening of the midface and a series of unflattering folds, a deepening of the nasolabial groove, marionette lines, and a less defined jaw line—jowls.

Cosmetic surgery and non-surgical treatments have moved beyond Hollywood and into our own backyards.

Blepharoplasty is one of the most popular cosmetic surgical procedures. In the age group 35–50, eyelid surgery was performed four times more frequently than facelifts. In the age group 51–64, eyelid surgery was performed twice as frequently as a facelift.

WHO IS HAVING EYELID SURGERY?	
AGES 19-34	10.0%
AGES 35-50	39.0%
AGES 51-64	41.9%
AGES 65+	8.7%
Source: ASAPS 2004	

The surgical approach to the eyelids is no longer simply about removal of skin and fat. It is about internal support, tendon tightening, fat repositioning, soft tissue augmentation, skin rejuvenation with collagen stimulation and resurfacing.

Blepharoplasty and eyelid rejuvenation have evolved into a completely new art form.

Our laser-assisted eyelid procedures can restore a youthful look to the upper eyelid, as well as improve the appearance of the lower eyelid area. Traditionally, fat was removed from below the eye to eliminate bags through an eyelid skin incision. About fifteen years ago we stopped performing skin incisions under the eyelashes since they had a tendency to pull the lower eyelid down, causing narrowing and rounding of the eye. About twelve years ago we began using the carbon dioxide laser to perform these procedures without cutting the lower eyelid skin. The carbon dioxide laser allowed us to perform this surgery without any bleeding.

The Concept of Facial Harmony

There are eighteen muscles that make our eyes blink approximately twenty times a minute, for a total of 12,000 daily movements.

Since the ideal goal in facial rejuvenation is restoring a youthful appearance while maintaining the harmony and balance of the face, a forehead lift, a surgical or non-surgical facelift, Botox® and filler facial reshaping may be recommended, depending on your age or degree of facial aging. Reviewing your high school yearbook pictures with you can be a great help when we decide the shape and fullness of your eyelids that we want to recreate. You will be evaluated. Since no two eyelids are exactly alike, we will design an individualized treatment plan for you.

Your eyes and eyelids are perpetually moving. The orbicularis muscles (eyelid sphincter muscles) close each eye. The levator and Müller's muscles open each eye. The frontalis muscle raises the eyebrow. The corrugator, procerus and orbicularis muscles depress the eyebrow. This constant motion inevitably changes skin tone and tissue elasticity. Frequent sun exposure not only affects the quality and texture of the skin, but increases wrinkling because of constant squinting.

What causes dark circles?

If your dark circles disappear when your photo is taken with a flash, then your dark circles are not really dark circles, but shadows from bulging fat.

DARK CIRCLES	
CAUSES	**CURES**
WRINKLES	Botulinum toxin, short chain poly-Peptide creams, CO2Cellulair™, Thermage Eye Tip
SKIN PIGMENT	Bleaching creams, chemical peels, CO2Cellulair™, laser resurfacing
VASCULAR POOLING	CO2Cellulair™
TEAR TROUGH	Restylane™, fat transposition
LOWER LID BAGS	CO2Cellulair™, blepharoplasty

Dark under eye circles can be caused by blood vessels or accumulated blood pooling showing through the thin eyelid skin. They are often visible around the eye contour because of the constant flow of blood, eye movement and skin transparency. They can also be caused by inherited pigment in the skin or darkening of skin pigment after recurrent inflammation or allergies. Dark circles can be caused by the shadows cast by bulging fat or lower lid bags. Puffiness and bags are caused by orbital fat that slides forward when the eyelid tissues are not firm enough to hold it back. This is usually an inherited trait, but is aggravated by aging. Any tendency for swelling or fluid retention will make the bags seem worse. Filling in the depressions with Restylane® may camouflage them and postpone the need for surgery.

Avoid rubbing your eyes constantly—it can accelerate the aging process and damage delicate eyelid skin.

Am I ready for eyelid surgery?

If you are contemplating eyelid surgery, you may benefit from learning how to evaluate your eyelid region as an Oculoplastic Surgeon would.

To evaluate your upper face, we examine you in both a scientific and an aesthetic manner to determine the most suitable treatment.

Even after you have had a good night's sleep, do people still comment that you look tired after you have been up for several hours?

When you are tired, your eyelids appear heavy and puffy, but when you awaken the puffiness is gone. As the eyelid ages and the eyelid and supportive tissue lose their elasticity, however, sleep alone will no longer make you look refreshed. When you are lying down or after having a salty meal, your eyelids tend to swell. Because the eyelid skin is so thin, fluid may accumulate in the lower lid and over the cheek bones, making bags appear worse. This swelling disappears after you arise and walk around. However, repeated episodes of this kind of swelling will eventually stretch out the eyelid tissues and they will not return to their youthful state.

Do other members of your family have droopy eyelids?

Look at your parents. Do they have heavy upper lids or lower lid bags? If so, your eyes may age in a similar way. Genetics play a huge role in all facets of aging, and eyelid drooping and bags tend to run in families.

Do you feel extra heaviness on your upper eyelids? When you lift the upper eyelid skin with your fingers, does it open your eyelid area up? Does the excess skin that falls above the eyelid crease have the texture of crepe paper?

When upper eyelid skin loses its elasticity, the fold tends to become heavy and to fall over the upper eyelid crease. This can leave no space for make-up. It can even block part of your peripheral vision. The loss of elasticity will affect the skin texture making it difficult for make-up to adhere to the skin. Trimming the excess upper lid fold will make the fold cleaner. Sculpting the upper lid fat will flatten the fold. Laser resurfacing will tighten the fold and smooth the skin.

Do you have horizontal creases across your forehead?

To counteract the effects of drooping upper eyelids, which create a shadow and block peripheral vision, muscles in the forehead involuntarily contract to raise the eyebrows and the eyelids. To compensate for extra skin around the eyelids, people often tend to elevate their eyebrows unconsciously, which can be the cause of deep lines and folds across the forehead area. When excess upper lid skin or a drooping upper lid either blocks the light entering the pupil or creates a shadow, the eye senses the constriction of the peripheral vision and signals the brain to raise the eyebrows.

Do your heavy upper eyelids make you tired?

Constant elevation of the eyebrows can give you headaches by the end of the day. Reading can make you very tired. The muscles get tired and ache like any other muscles. If your eyelids are heavy and drooping, the forehead frontalis muscle must work overtime to keep with pupils uncovered and to allow sufficient light to enter.

Eyelid skin may be blocking the visual field and consequently interfering with your peripheral vision. To check, gently lift your upper eyelids with your fingers to simulate the effects of upper eyelid surgery. Drooping eyelids create the effect of looking out of a window with the window shades half down. Because the forehead muscle (frontalis) is constantly working to raise the eyebrows and the upper lids, it may get tired like any other muscle. This may cause frontal headaches and these fatigued muscles' inability to continue to hold the eyelids up may be the reason the droopy lids are worse later in the day.

Do you have bags or puffiness under your eyes?

These are not really fatty deposits. The eyes sit in a bony cavity. Fat pockets around the eye act as protective shock absorbers. Either age or genetics cause a weakness in the tissue that holds the fat back behind the eye, then the fat falls forward, creating a bag. A loose or stretched lateral canthal tendon lowers the level of the lower lid and also causes horizontal narrowing of the eye, making it look smaller and rounder. This loose tendon also causes more folding of the lower eyelid skin, like sheets on a clothesline when the clothesline is loose. Allergies or salty foods can make bags look worse. If you have lower lid bags or looseness of the lower lid tendons, Botox® may accentuate the tendon looseness by relaxing the muscles that support the lower lid and camouflage the lower lid bags.

CHECK OFF ALL THAT APPLY

- [ ] My eyes are always in a shadow.
- [ ] My peripheral vision has gotten worse with age.
- [ ] Most evenings I have a forehead headache.
- [ ] I have no place to put my eye shadow.
- [ ] My upper eyelashes have disappeared and are covered by my upper lid skin.
- [ ] My eyes don't open.
- [ ] My eyes seem smaller.
- [ ] I need to raise my eyebrows to see.
- [ ] When I pick up the skin of my upper lids with my fingers, I can see better.
- [ ] My eyelid skin is wrinkled and looks like crepe paper.
- [ ] My eyes seem rounder, less almond-shaped.
- [ ] I have lower lid puffiness.
- [ ] I can see the white under my eyes.
- [ ] I have dark circles under my eyes.
- [ ] I have folds on my lower eyelids.
- [ ] I have bags on my cheeks.
- [ ] Salty food makes my eyelids puffy.

Monica's Upper Eyelid Surgery

Monica was contemplating upper eyelid surgery but was concerned about muscle and fat excision changing the shape of her eye and making her look too thin as she aged. We explained to her that the orbicularis muscle is partially removed in patients that have blepharospasm (uncontrollable eyelid muscle spasms) that do not respond to Botox®. Some surgeons may also remove this for cosmetic purposes, but we do not recommend it. Removing a strip of pretarsal orbicularis muscle and fat from the upper lid can make some patients look gaunt. Some surgeons have a standard routine that they follow that may work for some patients and not for others. That is why we individualize our surgical approach. We have an entire menu of surgical options. We have to analyze the patients' anatomy, examine their old photos, discuss their desires, and then make our choice of which procedures to use and how they should be performed. Some patients lose fat around their eyes as they age, making their eyes look deep and sunken. Others have fatty tissue prolapse, producing bagginess and heaviness. These conditions have to be managed differently. We informed Monica that it is sometimes reasonable to remove some muscle in the upper lid to create a better crease. However, we do not find this the case in the lower lid where we feel that this muscle is necessary to support the lower lid.

We removed some skin from Monica's upper lids and sculpted her upper lid fat by melting it with a carbon dioxide laser. We did not remove any orbicularis muscle from her upper lid. She was pleased with her natural result and felt that her eyelids were much less heavy.

CHAPTER 3

Brow Essentials

When you are young, your eyebrows sit in the right position and the forehead muscles do not have to work to keep them there. As you get older the tissues that support your eyebrows stretch and they start to droop.

There is a constant interplay between the position of the eyebrows, the muscles of the forehead, and the upper lid skin fold. As the tissues descend, they may even droop lower than the orbital bone above your eye (the superior orbital rim). This will cause your upper eyelids to collapse, making the skin fold heavier. Your body responds subconsciously by using your forehead muscles to raise your eyebrows and put them in the right position again, all of this constant forehead muscle activity will cause transverse (horizontal) creases across your forehead.

So now, what do we do? If we give you Botox® to your forehead muscle, all the horizontal folds will disappear and you will have a smooth forehead again, but you will not be able to hold your eyebrows in the right position and your upper eyelids will be heavy. This is when an eyebrow lift can help.

INNOVATIONS IN BROW LIFTING

We prefer a natural, minimally invasive approach. This will avoid a surprised, unnatural look with eyebrows that are in the middle of your forehead. The brow level and contour are obviously important. The eyebrows express many different emotions—surprise, anger, concern, sadness. Poorly positioned or shaped eyebrows may not convey what you really feel. The eyebrows are the frame for the eyes. There are many variations of brow lifts performed today.

Eyebrow lift through eyelid incision with the BZ Lift

This is our favorite technique because it is so minimally invasive. It is part of our patent-pending **BZ Lift** procedure. A subtle eyebrow lift or even just internal eyebrow stabilization is performed through an eyelid crease incision (just like an eye lift or blepharoplasty). And it is sometimes referred to as the trans-blepharoplasty internal brow suspension. This incision will allow us to remove fatty tissue or sagging upper eyelid skin at the same time if that is what you need. The procedure is simple and successful, especially if the brow droop mostly involves the outer part of the brow toward the ear. To make this procedure even more effective, one to two weeks before the surgery, we will treat the muscles that are pulling your eyebrow down with Botox® so that they will be relaxed and pull down less. Following the placement of your internal support suture, we will tighten your forehead tissues with Thermage®. This will give extra support to keep your eyebrow in the right place.

Small incision endoscopic brow lift

Although this is a very popular technique that has specific indications, we more often recommend a minimally invasive laser approach performed through an eyelift incision.

Change in brow shape may significantly change the facial expression. Elevating the brow too high may result in a surprised appearance. In such cases, the eye may dry or get irritated due to incomplete closure. These symptoms are similar to those occurring with excision of too much skin in an upper lid lift. If the brow is not raised enough, drooping will persist.

With brow lifting, the key is to find the right balance for every patient and to avoid the dreaded "deer in the head-lights" look.

OPEN BROW LIFT (CORONAL TECHNIQUE)

This technique was once the most frequently performed brow lifting procedure. It is still a very effective surgical option for cases of severe brow ptosis (drooping). In this era of minimally invasive techniques, many patients are alienated by the extensive incision and possible complications.

THREAD LIFTS

Another trend is the evolution of microscopic barbed sutures with tiny fingers that hold onto the tissues under the skin. While the new Contour Threadlift™ technique is gaining popularity, we are still evaluating exactly what place it may have in our menu of minimally invasive techniques. It is commonly used for elevating the soft tissues of the brows, midface, and neck and jowl area, and has a temporary effect of one to four years. It may very well supplement lifting and tissue tightening following Thermage® or Titan® treatments, in those areas that need additional support. The potential advantages of this technology are still evolving and dissolvable versions are barbed sutures are on being studied for use in facial rejuvenation.

ARCHERY—SHAPING THE BROW

The shape and contour of the eyebrows are critical to the overall appearance of the face. Not only do the brows represent facial expression, they are the frame for the eyes. They accentuate the beauty of the eyes. They need to have the proper relationship with the upper eyelids. Without the eyebrows in their appropriate position, upper eyelid surgery cannot be performed accurately. After the eyebrows have been put in the right place and given a shape that fits with your eyes and face and eyelids have been rejuvenated, we rejuvenate the eyebrows themselves. If there are hairs missing or the eyebrow hair is too thin, we can replace them with hair transplantation. If the eyebrow hair is too light or too sparse, micropigmentation—a delicate form of tattooing—can make the brow hairs appear denser and darker (see Chapter 7).

CHAPTER 4

Upper Eyelid Renewal

Now that we can understand eyelid anatomy more thoroughly, our concepts of beauty have changed, and we strive for a less operated look.

In the past many surgeons and patients viewed upper eyelid blepharoplasty as simply a procedure where excess skin and fat were removed from the eyelids. Technology has given us multiple options for achieving our end result. We can now not only improve eyelid appearance, but improve eyelid function and slow down the signs of eyelid aging all at the same time. Efficient and effective functional repair of the upper lid requires brow stabilization or elevation, correction of muscles that have slipped out of position, repositioning of the tear gland, and cutaneous laser resurfacing to tighten and smooth eyelid skin.

When we evaluate you for an upper eyelid blepharoplasty, and after we have determined your eyebrow position, we review your old photos to see what your upper eyelid fold looked like in your high school graduation picture. You may have had full upper lids even when you were a teenager. Not everyone has deep upper lids. So it may not be appropriate to give you deep upper lids. We will use your old pictures as a guide. In cases where the eyelid fold droops over the eyelashes and covers the eyelid margin, we will have to remove some skin. If your upper lid skin is only slightly loose, we may perform a light laser resurfacing without removing any tissue. In many cases we do both; removing the extra skin and tightening the remaining skin with a laser. This will give you the most natural result with the longest lasting effect—a clean upper lid crease and tighter, smoother upper lid skin with renewed elasticity. The upper lid has a younger appearance, and the tissues are rejuvenated following CO2Cellulair™, Thermage Eye Tip, or laser resurfacing.

NON-SURGICAL UPPER EYELID REJUVENATION	
PROBLEM	**SOLUTION**
DROOPY BROW	Botulinum toxin + Thermage brow Lift – BZ Lift
HEAVY EYELID SKIN	Thermage Eye Tip, CO2Cellulair™, Laser resurfacing
CREPE-LIKE SKIN TEXTURE	Chemical peels, CO2Cellulair™, Thermage Eye Tip, Laser resurfacing

We cannot stop the aging process entirely, but we can turn back the clock and slow it down.

Sometimes the upper lid appears droopy because one of the muscles that opens the eye is either not working properly or has shifted out of position. The levator muscle's tendon can be separated from its normal location as a result of excessive eye or eyelid rubbing, removal, insertion, or extensive manipulation of contact lens (especially hard contact lens), previous eye or eyelid surgery; and recurrent eyelid swelling because of allergy, eye, or eyelid infections. This muscle separation and eyelid drooping can even be more prominent when you are looking down and can interfere with your reading. We often repair this muscle at the time we are performing an upper eyelid blepharoplasty. The tendon of the muscle (aponeurosis) can have slipped, it can be thinned or completely degenerated. We will describe the surgical procedure to repair a droopy eyelid in the section on ptosis correction.

On the day of surgery, we discuss the procedures to be performed and mark the eyelids with a surgical marking pen, to make sure that we are doing exactly what you want us to do. We can do a great job technically, but if it is not what you wanted, none of us will be pleased. The blepharoplasty is performed in our office operating room with local anesthesia and intravenous sedation given by our board certified anesthesiologist. While you are taking a short nap, your eyelids will be numbed. The upper eyelid skin incision is designed to fit into your natural lid crease. We use a carbon dioxide laser to make the incisions to seal the blood vessels as it cuts, reducing the chance of bleeding and bruising. The excess skin is removed. The excess fatty tissue in the upper eyelid exposes itself by bulging forward. Rather than cutting the fat, we melt it with the carbon dioxide laser. This method allows us to literally sculpt the fat without any bleeding. We close the incision with individual tiny sutures. Even though this suture technique takes a few extra minutes, it gives the wound closure extra strength. These sutures are left in place for five to seven days, then they are removed in the office. Many of our patients travel for surgery so we can use dissolvable stitches that fall out by themselves in about one week.

Laser incisional blepharoplasty and ptosis repair with the carbon dioxide laser allows us to perform the surgery in a bloodless field which reduces the operative time. Less trauma to the delicate eyelid tissues translates to a faster return to your normal activities.

PTOSIS REPAIR FOR DROOPY UPPER EYELID

Blepharoptosis repair (repair of a drooping eyelid) involves reinserting the levator muscle tendon to its proper position so that it can elevate the eyelid margin to where it belongs. We do this through a blepharoplasty incision in the upper lid crease, and we often perform this correction at the time of blepharoplasty. To ensure that we have put your muscle in the correct position and that your eyes open equally, we will ask you to open and close your eyes so we can watch the muscle move and see exactly where we should put it. Sometimes we have you sit up during the surgery to match the lid levels. Tiny stitches secure the levator aponeurosis and close the skin, creating a normal crease.

The elevation of the eyelid will often be immediately noticeable, though in some cases bruising and swelling will obscure it. Most of the swelling and bruising is gone in three to four days. Cold packs are applied to the operated eyelid as often as is comfortable for the first 48 hours following surgery. Antibiotic ointment is applied to the stitches twice daily. You will continue taking Arnica Montana pellets under your tongue four times a day until the swelling is gone. Your stitches will be removed in one week or, if you have absorbable stitches, they will fall out by themselves.

ETHNIC EYELID DIFFERENCES

Concepts of beauty differ from one country to the next, and people from different races have varying eyelid structures.

The anatomy of the Asian eyelid and African and African-American eyelid is different from the anatomy of the Caucasian eyelid. The eyelids of each ethnic background have different characteristics—not only diverse amounts of pigment, but also different skin thickness, skin and muscle insertions, location and amount of fatty tissue, healing tendencies, and surrounding bony structure.

THE ASIAN EYELID

The Asian eyelid is dramatically different from the Caucasian eyelid. The Asian eyelid has more subcutaneous fat, making a fuller upper eyelid, and is often without a lid crease. The levator muscle inserts lower on the eyelid, making a lower lid crease, sometimes so low that it is not perceived. In some cases there is no lid crease at all. This is called the "single eyelid" and is differentiated from an eyelid with a lid crease or a "double eyelid." Converting a single eyelid to a double eyelid is a commonly performed procedure where a small strip of skin and muscle is removed and sutures are used to attach the skin to the underlying muscle to make a crease.

Some surgical techniques produce deep, immobile creases that persist even when your eyes are closed. We prefer a technique that produces a more natural result—where the crease is not too deep and naturally disappears when your eye is closed.

The Upper Lid Crease

The eyelid crease is an exceptionally important structure for all of our patients. The lid crease is even more important for our Asian patients because crease level and contour has a specific ethnic character. Different Asian countries have diverse concepts of beauty. Some countries value the lower lid crease, while others prefer a slightly higher lid crease. We try to modify eyelids with great subtlety, elevating the lid crease slightly and avoiding making the crease too deep, and even slightly changing the direction of the outside corner of the eye, to preserve natural ethnic characteristics.

In Western culture, an upper eyelid is generally considered attractive if it lacks excessive skin and fat, possesses a reasonably well-defined and high crease, and displays at least some platform of exposed skin between the crease and the eyelashes. Likewise, a well-contoured lower eyelid free of bulging fat projects an image of youth, energy, and rest.

The Asian eyelid crease often is closer to the eyelashes, not as deep, and may be incomplete, irregular, or broken into multiple creases. In about half of Asian patients, there is little or even no crease at all. In some cases, the creases on the two sides are not symmetric.

The absence of a defined crease—the single lid—makes the opening between the eyelids appear narrower than it really is. A double lid, that is a lid with a crease that divides the eyelid into two visual parts, makes the same size opening appear wider. The Asian eyelid may also appear fuller because subcutaneous fat continues down to the upper lid lashes and also extends to the brow, creating a flat eyelid contour.

By far, the primary concern in the majority of Asian patients seeking blepharoplasty is the final position and shape of the upper eyelid crease.

ISSUES IN ASIAN BLEPHAROPLASTY

• **SHAPE**—While a typical non-Asian upper eyelid crease tends to be highest in the middle position of the eyelid and taper lower at each end, such a "semilunar" shape many not appear natural on your face. An attractive Asian crease will either run parallel to the eyelid margin throughout its entire course or dip slightly downward as the nose is approached.

• **HEIGHT**—While a typical Occidental female crease may sit 10 mm above the margin of the lid, in Asian patients the crease will appear more "natural" at a lower height ranging from 2 to 5 mm.

• **CONTINUITY**—Incomplete creases may be enhanced without changing the shape or height, by "completing" the crease so that it runs continuously. Multiple poorly-defined creases may be converted into one dominant crease.

Attempting to achieve too radical a transformation of the pre-existing anatomy is generally unwise and may result in eyelids that look unnatural or mismatched to the rest of the face. To avoid an inappropriate or disappointing result, the steps of any eyelid operation may be adjusted to take into account the variations in your anatomy as well as your goals.

Upper Lid Asian Blepharoplasty

The position of the proposed new crease (you will be looking in the mirror to make sure that we put it exactly where you want it) is marked with a pen on your eyelid skin and overlies the upper border of the tarsal plate (usually about 5 to 8 mm above the lashes). Because Asian skin heals differently than Caucasian skin, we use a scalpel instead of the carbon dioxide laser to cut the skin. The incision may be tapered into the epicanthal fold towards the nose (if desired) and/or flared upwards at its outer end (if desired).

A small strip of skin above this initial incision is excised using the carbon dioxide laser. The incision is carried deeper into the eyelid through the orbicularis muscle and orbital septum, and the orbital fat is exposed. Small strips of muscle and orbital septum are removed, and a small amount of fat can be vaporized with the laser.

Suture closure of the skin employs a "deep-fixation" technique in which the needle engages the levator aponeurosis near the top of the tarsal plate in multiple spots along the length of the incision, thus creating an attachment between the aponeurosis and the tissue just below the skin. The crease that is created is a result of both tissue removal and deep-fixation. This type of fixation creates a much more natural crease than those created with "full thickness" sutures that come all the way through your eyelid. Surgery performed through a skin incision creates a permanent crease.

Even if your skin is not very dark, laser resurfacing can take longer to heal. There will invariably be a period of transient hyperpigmentation that will need to be treated with retinol, hydroquinone, and topical cortisone. We often prefer to treat Asian eyelid skin with light chemical peels instead of laser resurfacing.

Full Thickness Suture Approach to the Asian Upper Eyelid

Less invasive techniques have been described that involve placement of sutures into and through the eyelid without making a skin incision. The sutures cause tissue compression and temporary internal inflammation, which create an internal scar that holds the crease in place.

Because a non-incisional approach does not allow for the removal of any eyelid tissue, the major impediments to crease formation—the existence of subcutaneous fat and lack of internal adhesions—are not addressed and the crease that is formed after a non-incisional approach looks less natural (for instance, the crease is present whether your eyelid is open or closed) and will disappear with time. We do not use the suture approach because the crease that is created is less natural and usually does not give a permanent result.

Epicanthoplasty

Eliminating or revising the epicanthal fold can be difficult because of its location in the highly visible and easily distorted tissues of the multi-contoured area between the nose and eye. We have succeeded in achieving subtle, natural modifications of the epicanthal fold by incorporating the fold into a new lid crease. We avoid complicated procedures that use multiple incisions and skin flaps, which may result in unacceptable scarring.

UPPER EYELID SURGERY IN PATIENTS OF AFRICAN DESCENT

Patients of African descent not only have a different skin type and different healing characteristics, but they have a different shape to their orbital bones—the bones surrounding the eye. This makes eyelid puffiness and prominent eyes more common and requires different surgical approaches if you want to modify these characteristics.

Because your orbital bones have a different shape and a shallower orbital bony cavity, all of the structures within your orbit, including the eyeball, may be pushed forward. In your upper lid this includes fat that may make your upper lid heavy and the lacrimal gland that will make the outside part of your upper lid heavy as well.

Due to the skin's tendency for darkening and lightening we use a scalpel instead of the carbon dioxide laser to perform the skin incisions for your upper eyelid blepharoplasty. We still use the laser to melt the excess fat and to sculpt your upper lid, giving it a more defined contour. When we encounter your lacrimal gland in the outside portion of your upper lid, we do not melt it. We secure it in its proper position behind the superior orbital rim with a permanent suture. This holds the gland where is belongs and reduces the heaviness of your upper lid.

The use of resurfacing lasers on darker skin types usually produces at least a temporary period of hyperpigmentation. However, the more serious problem is one of permanent hypopigmentation or skin lightening. We have used lasers to resurface eyelids with dark skin and have achieved impressive results, but only using lower power settings. As an alternative, we often recommend light TCA peels.

Keloids on the eyelids are rarely a problem, even if there is a tendency to get keloids on other areas of your body. Perhaps because the eyelid skin is so thin, the eyelids are a protected area.

How We Do It

Achieving excellent results with eyelid surgery involves a delicate touch and great attention to the finest details.

Before our anesthesiologist administers sedatives, we will make the surgical markings on your eyelids while you are sitting upright. We may ask you to open and close your eyelids. To protect you from the bright operating room lights, we will place topical anesthetic eye drops in your eyes and then a protective contact lens will be placed in front of each eye.

We always operate on the upper eyelids first and then the lower eyelids. With our current procedure, using the CO_2 lasers to melt the fat, there is no pulling. We use this laser to accurately sculpt the fat without any bleeding. If you feel any discomfort, you can ask the anesthesiologist for additional sedation or we can administer local injections into the eyelid tissues. Our team will do everything to make you comfortable to make your surgical experience pleasant.

CHAPTER 5

Revitalizing the Lower Lids

Our approach to lower lid rejuvenation is more physiologic, less traumatic, minimally invasive, and reduces complications.

Our years of experience correcting eyelids that have been pulled and stretched out of place from unexpected scarring, improperly performed procedures, or just from having too much surgery have convinced us not to cut the skin of the lower eyelid when performing cosmetic surgery.

Our philosophy is very straightforward. We remove the fat (or shift it from where it is bulging to where there is an indentation) from the inside of the eyelid without cutting the eyelid skin (transconjunctival approach), tighten the tendon if it is loose, and use a laser to make the skin tighter and smoother. We use Botox® to relax the muscles before surgery and laser resurfacing. Following the surgery, we use a variety of fillers to treat depressions around the orbital bones.

The simplest way to think of the lower lid support system is to imagine a hammock hanging between two trees.

The equivalent of the main body of the hammock would be a thin cartilage-like structure that gives shape to the eyelid and is known as the tarsus or tarsal plate. The tarsal plate is connected to the orbital rim of bone (the two trees) by a tendon on each side (the connecting ends of the hammock), known as the medial canthal tendon (on the side towards the nose) and the lateral canthal tendon (on the side towards the temple). This lower lid support system is critical to the stability of the lower lid. If the medial and lateral canthal tendons are loose, the lower lid margin drops away from the eye; this is called an ectropion. If the medial and lateral canthal tendons are loose, sometimes the lower lid margin and the eyelashes may turn towards the eye and rub on the cornea, causing severe discomfort; this is called an entropion. If a transcutaneous lower lid blepharoplasty has been performed and lower eyelid skin has been removed, the lower eyelid can be pulled down towards the cheek and the eye will not close completely; called lower lid retraction.

Tightening the lateral canthal tendon can prevent and also correct lower lid ectropion, entropion, and retraction. For this reason we always tighten a loose lateral canthal tendon when we are performing a cosmetic lower lid blepharoplasty. To prevent any displacement of the lower eyelid, we always tighten the lateral canthal tendon before we perform lower eyelid skin resurfacing. This will prevent the new, tight skin from pulling the lower lid down or away from the eye. We place a permanent stitch beneath the skin through the tendon and attach it to the lateral orbital bony rim. This is performed through two tiny incisions—one at the outside end of the lower lid and one at the outside end of the upper eyelid crease.

A similar basic support system exists in the upper lid. The orbital septum is a fibrous membrane that can be thought of as holding back the fat that fills the eye socket and cushions the eyeball. In the lower eyelid, the orbital septum connects to the tarsus and extends all the way to rim of bone beneath the eye. In the upper lid, the orbital septum connects very near the top of the tarsal plate and extends all the way to the rim of bone at the eyebrow.

Eyelid Fat

Think of the upper eyelid fat as consisting of two pockets: a long thin middle fat pocket and a globular nasal fat pocket. While, the lower eyelid fat has three pockets, the nasal, middle, and temporal fat pockets. If the orbital septum is stripped away, the eyelid fat will be exposed. The upper eyelid fat lies just in front of the levator aponeurosis. Eyelid fat is really an extension of the same orbital fat that fills the entire socket.

Sculpting and Repositioning Fat

We use the carbon dioxide laser to open the inner mucous membrane lining of the eyelid—the conjunctiva. The laser seals the blood vessels as it opens the conjunctiva, the fat bulges forward, and we melt the fat, sculpting it with the laser. If there are depressed areas in the eyelid, instead of vaporizing the fat completely, we move it into the indented areas and put in a stitch to hold the transposed fat in place against the skin. CO2Cellulair™ can also be used to improve the appearance of some buldging fat and the Thermage eye tip can tighten lower lid skin.

Deeper Eyelid

Eyelid fat sits just in front of the tendons of the main opening muscles and tendons (known also as the "retractors") of the eyelids. The main opening muscle/tendon system in the upper eyelid is the levator muscle or aponeurosis. Small strands of tissue extending from the levator aponeurosis help to create the upper eyelid crease.

The main opening muscle/tendon system in the lower eyelid is called the capsulopalpebral fascia. The deepest layers of the upper eyelid consist of a smaller retractor muscle (Müller's muscle) which helps open the upper lid and pull down the lower lid. The lining of the inside of the eyelid is a mucous membrane called the conjunctiva.

Lower Lid Asian Blepharoplasty

Lower lid Asian blepharoplasty has to be performed differently than common lower lid blepharoplasty techniques. Your surgery will still be performed from the inside of your lower lid—to avoid cutting the skin—but the fat has to sculpted very carefully to avoid making the lid too deep. The fat must be sculpted so that the front surface of the eyelid has a smooth relationship to the cheek bone and does not leave an indentation between the lower eyelid and the cheekbone. Tightening the outside (lateral canthal) tendon is done delicately to preserve the precise angle. If the lower lid muscle that is just in front of the lashes, we flatten it with Botox® rather than cutting the skin.

The Lower Epicanthal Fold

There can also be a lower epicanthal fold that extends from the lower eyelid crease to the side of the nose. The fold can be large or small and can be softened by incorporating it into the eyelid form.

Vertical Eyelashes

The same attachments from the muscle to the eyelid skin that create the upper eyelid crease and support the upper lid lashes, also support the projection of the lower lid lashes. Because the Asian eyelid lacks these supportive attachments, the lashes do not slope gently away from the eye. Rather they are more vertically directed and sometimes can irritate the cornea. If these lashes are irritating the cornea, we rotate them by creating new internal eyelid muscle and skin attachments.

Lower Eyelid Blepharoplasty in Patients of African Descent

Because of the relationship between the eyelids and your orbital bones, the eyes may be prominent, the white of the eyes may be visible below the cornea, the lower eyelid margins may droop and the lower lid fat may push forward and create bags. Using the carbon dioxide laser to sculpt the fat from the inside of the eyelids (without cutting skin) and to tighten and raise the outside corner supportive tendons (lateral canthal tendon) makes this procedure more effective, without creating any eyelid scars or keloids.

The Eye Socket

The eye is protected by the bony orbit. You can feel the orbital rims above, below, and to the sides of the eye. These bones are strong. Inside the orbit, fat pockets cushion and protect the eye, the optic nerve, and the muscles that move the eyes in all directions. The bones inside the orbit are not as strong as the rims. They can be fractured easily, entrapping eye muscles and causing double vision.

RESTORING THE PERIORBITAL AREA

Lower eyelid blepharoplasty procedures sculpt and reposition bulging fat from under the eye. Skin that is wrinkled and lax, that appears to be excessive, is supported by tightening the lateral canthal tendon and is treated with chemical peels and laser resurfacing. We avoid the traditional complications of lower lid blepharoplasty by not cutting and removing skin.

We achieve our goals by melting and repositioning fat through a conjunctival incision on the inside of the eyelid to avoid lower eyelid scarring. This technique alone may be adequate to improve the eyelids in young patients. Through a tiny skin incision just below the eyelashes and at the outside of the eyelid, the lower eyelid supportive lateral canthal tendon is tightened with a permanent suture.

Tightening of the eyelid ligaments at the corner of the eye, the lower arm of the lateral canthal tendon is necessary to support the eyelid. A horizontally loose eyelid will sag much like a loose clothesline with the weight of only a few clothes if the clothesline is not properly supported. The lateral canthopexy tightens and stabilizes the lower eyelid.

Once the support of your lower lid has been stabilized and the eyelid contour adjusted and smoothed, the periorbital skin can be relaxed with Botox® and rejuvenated with ablative and non-ablative lasers and chemical peels.

FAT REMOVAL

By removing hills and valleys, eyelid shadows are decreased.

When the orbital fat that surrounds the eye bulges forward, it creates elevations, shadows and dark circles under the eye. Bulging fat, by creating shadows, accentuates dark skin pigmentation—a problem that is only partially resolved by blepharoplasty. The pigment in the skin is not specifically improved by blepharoplasty. We can predict whose dark circles will be improved by blepharoplasty by taking a flash photograph before surgery. If the bags and circles disappear in the photographic image, that is confirmation that the skin itself is not pigmented. If only fat is protruding, which is the case in younger patients, no skin tightening is necessary.

Dark Circles

Lower lid dark circles may be caused by skin pigmentation, shadows, or pooled blood and many blood vessels that show through the transparent lower lid skin. Sculpting the lower lid fat pockets will eliminate the shadows. Laser resurfacing of the lower eyelid skin will eliminate dark pigmentation, and by creating new collagen, create thicker skin and a visual barrier obscuring the dark blood vessels under the skin.

CO2Cellulair™ uses small amounts of carbon dioxide gas to trick your body into thinking that there is not enough oxygen. And the response is an increase in oxygen and blood flow to the areas treated. We have studied this technique extensively, published our findings and found that this creates an impressive improvement in the quality, texture, contour, and pigmentation of eyelid skin. Small amounts of carbon dioxide gas are injected just under the eyelid skin. The eyelid skin remains inflated for three to five minutes. The downtime is under five minutes! The treatment is repeated once a week for four weeks. Improvement begins after one treatment and improves each week.

The Procedure

We make a conjunctival incision (the conjunctiva is the clear layer that "connects" the eyelid to the eyeball) on the inside of the lower eyelid. The risk of causing lower eyelid pull down or inferior scleral show (exposed white underneath the iris) is reduced with this method. This is the big advantage of the transconjunctival approach over the traditional blepharoplasty that is performed through a skin incision.

After the conjunctiva is opened and the small fibers that hold the fat back are vaporized, the fat will bulge forward and we then melt it, sealing blood vessels at the same time so that there is no bleeding or bruising. If there are areas of depressions, the bulging fat is moved into the depressed areas and held in place with absorbable sutures. The conjunctiva is not sutured. At the end of the procedure we smooth the eyelid skin and shift all the tissues gently back into their natural position.

REPLACING YOUTHFUL FULLNESS

Lower eyelid blepharoplasty is not about removing fat. It is about giving the lower eyelids a smooth contour and preserving a youthful fullness.

The trend with lower eyelid surgery is restoration instead of removal. In fact, lower eyelids that have had too much fat removed make you look older. We use the transconjunctival approach to shift fat from the areas where there is too much to the areas where there is not enough. When there is not enough fat to move around, we use Restylane® and Perlane® to fill in depressions like the tear trough deformity.

RESTORING EYELASH FULLNESS, COLOR, AND CONTOUR

Micropigmentation of the lower lid lashes will restore youthful, attractive fullness. Single follicle hair transplantation is not as useful for rejuvenating the lower lid as it is for the upper lid because if the lashes grow against the cornea, they can be very irritating.

CHAPTER 6

Eyelid Restoration — Correcting the Effects of Previous Surgery & Aging

"The real voyage of discovery consists not in seeking new landscapes but having new eyes."—Marcel Proust

Correcting the complications of unsatisfactory eyelid surgeries is delicate work that requires extreme patience and a light hand.

For years we have been chosen to correct the complications of unfortunate eyelid surgeries. This is tricky because the eyelid tissues are delicate and have to function perfectly, and because patients who have had complications of previous eyelid surgery are often angry and afraid. They are afraid that the situation could be made worse, or that we will not be able to fix their problem. Our first task is to let patients know that we care, that we may have seen even worse problems, and that we will do everything that we can to make them look and feel better.

The eyelids blink many times a minute and have to wipe away and refresh tears from the delicate corneal surface. The eyelids and the front of the eye are in constant and intimate contact. Eyelid movement and eyelid contact with the eye have to be perfect. By understanding the eyelid anatomy and how the eyelids work, we can tighten and support the tissues where support is needed and add extra tissue when extra tissue is needed. We can graft skin from the other eyelid or from behind the ear. We can even borrow tissue from the inside of the upper lid, where the donor site is not felt or seen.

Our years of experience as eyelid plastic and reconstructive surgeons have given us the confidence and ability to find creative ways to make your eyelids work better.

REMEDIES FOR COMPLICATIONS FROM EYELID SURGERY	
THE UPPER LIDS	Difficulty closing eyelids: **Release of internal scar tissue** Lids will lag (not move enough) when you look down: **Add extra skin** Eyelashes may be pulled away from the eye: **Rotate lashes** Brows pull down: **Release and elevate brows** Upper lids look heavy: **Brow lift** Upper lid droops and not open all the way: **Repair eyelid opening muscle (levator aponeurosis)** Deep upper lids may look older rather than younger: **Fill with Restylane**
THE LOWER LIDS	Lower lid pulls too low: **Tendon tightening; release internal scarring** Horizontal narrowing of eye: **Tendon tightening** Lower eyelid pulled out (ectropion): **Add extra skin; tighten tendon** Tearing: **Rotate tear drain** Wrinkling: **Tendon tightening; laser resurfacing** Bulges: **Laser fat sculpting** Hollow eyelids: **Reposition fat**
DRY EYE	Inadequate eyelid closure: **Add extra skin; tighten tendon**
TEARING	Inadequate eyelid closure: **Add extra skin; tighten tendon** Malposition of tear drains: **Rotate and reposition tear drain**

The Upper Lids

If too much skin is removed from the upper lids, the eyelids may not close properly, and they will lag (not move enough) when you look down and the eyelashes may even be pulled away from the eye. This is repaired by adding skin, usually taken from behind the ear where there is a good match in skin texture and color; it is not too thick or sun damaged.

If your brows were drooping before your blepharoplasty and they were not supported during the procedure, then they will be pulled down after the surgery and your upper lids will still look heavy. To repair this, skin may have to be added to the upper lids before the brow can be lifted and supported.

If the muscle that opens your upper lid (levator aponeurosis) is damaged during your surgery (during the removal of fat), your upper lid will droop and not open all the way. This can be fixed by reattaching the muscle to its proper position.

If your upper lids are still heavy after surgery, a little more skin or a little more fat may have to be removed to achieve your desired result. You can always have more tissue removed, so it is better to strive for a natural, understated result.

If your upper lids are too deep or too hollow after your surgery, this can make you look older rather than younger. Filling in deep upper lids can be done with fat, Restylane® or Perlane®, but it is an inexact art form.

CO2CELLULAIR™

• Tiny needle injects small amounts of carbon dioxide gas.

• Procedure takes minutes (longer for larger areas).

• For eyelids: reduces fine lines, dark pigmentation, dark circles from poor circulation, puffiness; results begin after first treatment, improve with 4 - 5 treatments, one week apart.

• For arms abdomen, buttocks: 6 - 9 treatments, as often as twice a week; reduces fat, tightens skin.

The Lower Lids

We gave up performing traditional lower lid blepharoplasty a dozen years ago, and now we never cut the lower lid skin.

The most frequent complications that we see among the patients that are sent to us involve lower eyelid surgery. Cutting the lower eyelid skin is the main reason for these complications. Even if too much skin is not removed, the simple act of cutting the lower eyelid skin can lead to internal scarring that may change the shape of the eye or pull the lower lid too low. Avoiding incisions of the lower eyelid skin and recognizing any laxity or looseness of the supportive lateral canthal tendon, can avoid complications. We feel that almost all patients can have a wonderful result by removing bulging fat from the inside of the lid (transconjunctival approach), tightening the support tendon (lateral canthal tendon) when there is laxity, and resurfacing the skin with peels and lasers when necessary.

If your lower lid is pulled too low and the lid is loose, then tightening the supportive tendon will do the job. If your lower lid is pulled too low and the lid is tight, then you will need release of the scar tissue that is under the skin. We can usually do this from the inside of the eyelid without cutting the skin, internal support with a graft taken from the inside of the upper lid, and then tightening of the tendon. It is helpful to correct this as soon as possible because the longer that the eyelid is pulled down, the more the supportive tendon is stretched and the looser the eyelid will become.

If the inside lining of the eyelid is exposed and red (ectropion), then too much skin has been removed. This can usually be corrected by tightening the supportive tendon, but sometimes skin will have to be added to the lower eyelid as well.

If your eye is tearing and is bothered by light, your eyelids are probably not closing completely and your cornea is drying out. This can be fixed by tightening the supportive tendon, but extreme cases may need skin grafts for correction. If your eye is tearing, but it is not bothered by light, it may be that too much skin has been removed and your tear drain has been pulled out of position. If this malposition is slight, a small procedure on the inside of the eyelid, rotating the tear drain can fix the problem. If the malposition is severe, tendon tightening and skin grafting may be necessary.

If your lower eyelid skin is wrinkled after the fat bags have been removed, this does not mean that you need skin removed. It means that your skin texture and resilience needs correction. This is best accomplished with botulinum toxin to relax the muscles under the skin and skin resurfacing with peels, CO2Cellulair™, lasers or tightening with the Thermage eye tip or lasers.

If there are still bulges after surgery, there may be some fat left that needs sculpting. The transconjunctival approach (from the inside of the lower eyelid) is ideal for secondary lower eyelid re-operations. Because the skin is not cut, there is minimal scar tissue formed to pull the eyelid out of place and any remaining bulging fat can be easily vaporized with the carbon dioxide laser.

If there are some areas in the lower lid that are bulging and other areas that are indented, this can indicate that too much fat has been removed in some areas and not enough in other areas. Through the transconjunctival approach fat can be shifted into the indented areas, filling them out and creating a smoother eyelid contour.

What can be done for hollow eyelids?

Repositioning of fat works very well. But if there is not enough, then adding fat or fillers to the lower eyelid can be tricky, but it is the only solution that we have.

What about bleeding?

There are some possible complications of eyelid surgery that are serious and potentially vision threatening. Bleeding is the most serious. The fat pads that surround the eye have many blood vessels tucked inside of them. The traditional technique of cutting fat after it has been clamped and cauterized is traumatic to the delicate tissue around the eye, but it is effective in preventing bleeding in most cases. In fact only about one in 10,000 patients have bleeding following blepharoplasty. Although some bruising is common, severe bleeding that can cause loss of vision is exceptionally rare. High blood pressure can cause blood vessels to open and bleeding to occur several hours after surgery. The signs of severe bleeding include eye pain, an eye that feels very tight, and darkening of vision. If this occurs, the incisions have to be opened and the blood vessels sealed.

Using the carbon dioxide laser further reduces the possibility of any bleeding as it seals blood vessels as it cuts. The carbon dioxide is particularly effective in melting fatty tissue and sealing the blood vessels within the fat simultaneously.

DRY EYES

After eyelid surgery it may be necessary to use topical lubricants (over-the-counter artificial tear drops) temporarily for a few days and sometimes for several weeks because the eyelids are swollen and not closing completely. If everything goes smoothly, the need for tears should ultimately not be more frequent after surgery than it was before. An uncomplicated blepharoplasty will not worsen symptoms of a dry eye. In fact, by tightening the eyelid tendon, often the symptoms of dry eye are improved after eyelid surgery.

WHAT TO EXPECT AFTER SURGERY

Because of stiffness of the eyelids during the first two weeks after surgery, there is a decreased upper lid blink which leads to greater evaporation of tears, and relative dryness of the eyes. This may give you a feeling of grittiness or foreign body sensation. The eye may tear and be slightly red. The eyelids will be swollen, especially during the first three to four days after the surgery. Vision will be blurry during these first days after surgery because of the swelling, tearing, and the antibiotic ointment that you will be applying to the eye. You can watch TV and use your computer, but reading will be somewhat challenging during this period. These symptoms will improve dramatically after the first four days.

Surgeries to correct previous complications do take longer to heal. Redness and swelling also can take longer to fade.

Dry Eye Relief

Over-the-counter tear drops will relieve the symptoms of your dry eyes. Use tear drops three to four times a day, or even more frequently if you need them. In rare cases, an ointment, such as Refresh PM (Allergan), is recommended at bedtime. Tears without preservatives may be used in disposable small vials every hour while awake. Avoid touching your eye with the drop dispenser. Try different types of artificial tears for several days to find which drops give you the greatest relief. Refrigerated artificial tears can be extremely soothing.

BEAUTIFEYE TIP: Have your spouse or significant other check while you are sleeping to see if your eyes are open.

If your eyes are irritated, crusty, and stuck together when you wake up in the morning then they probably are slightly open when you are sleeping. If your nighttime ointment makes you blurry in the morning, you can try one of the thicker eye drops such as Celluvisc® (Allergan) instead.

How to use eye drops:

The drops should be placed in the space between the upper and lower eyelids on the side of the nose. Always wash your hands and read the label before using. It is only necessary that the drop hit the eyelashes to enter the eye. Only one drop in the eye is necessary; more than one drop will not have any greater effect. To prevent injury and contamination, the container of the medication should not touch the eye. If you have trouble getting the drops into your eye, lie back flat, close your eyes, place two drops on the side of your eye next to your nose, then open your eyes. The eye drops will flow into your eyes.

Dry eye also causes light sensitivity. Dark glasses with side panels or shields that keep light out of the eye and prevent wind from irritating the eyes are helpful. The eyes should be shielded from the direct blow of air conditioners, fans, and forced air heater both within the car and at home.

After droopy eyelid (blepharoptosis) repair, the eye is open more and more of the eye is exposed. More tears evaporate. If you have severe dry eye, a punctal plug will make you feel better. This tiny plastic plug (a miniature version of a bathtub plug) is inserted into the opening of the tear drain, on the edge of the eyelid near the nose, to decrease tear drainage. This procedure effectively retains tears that you have and lessens your symptoms. A trial of an absorbable collagen plug, which lasts a few days, usually predicts the relief that may occur with the more long-lasting silicone plugs.

ALL ABOUT TEARS

Tears are not just water. They are composed of three layers, the middle layer is liquid—most like water—and the outer layer is oily to keep the liquid tears from evaporating.

Tiny glands, located in the surface tissue on the white of the eye and lining the eyelids, constantly produce a baseline level of tears to keep our eyes comfortable and lubricated. The lacrimal gland, a large gland located behind the upper eyelid and below the outside of the brow bone, responds to emotion or eye irritation by producing larger quantities of tears.

Excess tears well up in the eye because too many tears are produced or, because the tears are not draining properly. Excess tears give the eye a moist appearance, and can collect along the border of the lower lid and overflow onto the cheek.

The tears of each eye drain into a tiny opening in each lid near the nose called a punctum and flow through a small canal into the lacrimal sac and down the nasolacrimal duct into the nose. This is why our noses run when we cry, since excess tears reach the nose through the normal tear drainage system.

Excessive tearing is basically a plumbing problem.

Tearing can result from injuries, birth defects (incomplete formation of the tear drains), and infections. Abnormal lid positions, an inturned eyelash, wind exposure, yawning, glaucoma, certain drugs, or eyestrain can also stimulate excessive tearing. When the eyelids are too lax, they are an ineffective lacrimal pump and do not move the tears effectively into the lacrimal drainage system.

Tearing is a vicious cycle. Patients with a dry eye often complain of tearing, which is known as epiphora, where there is an overflow of tearing even though the underlying problem is dry eyes. If you have dry eyes, you may not have enough liquid tears, so the eyelids produce more mucoid tears to compensate, which makes you teary.

A thorough examination is necessary to determine the cause of excessive tearing. A Schirmer Test is used to measure baseline tear production. We also check the small openings on the upper and lower eyelid margin near the nose, called the puncta, to make sure that they are not blocked, or covered with a membrane.

The best treatment depends on the cause. If the problem is dry eyes, artificial tear replacement or even closure of the tear drainage openings may be helpful. For example, if the cause is an inturned eyelash entropion, the offending eyelash is removed or the eyelid position is corrected. Abnormalities of the eyelid may require surgery. If the tear drainage system is blocked, recurrent infections can become a problem and surgery to open or bypass the blockage may be necessary. It may be necessary to make a new tear drain—an additional opening from the lacrimal sac into the nose, a procedure known as a dacryocystorhinostomy or DCR.

BLEPHARITIS

Blepharitis is an inflammation of the eyelids. Several rows of oil glands run along the rims or margins of the eyelids in the area where the lashes begin. When these glands become irritated or inflamed, they produce extra oily, greasy material that becomes deposited on the eyelid margins and eyelashes and may get into the eye. The pores of the oil glands may also become plugged up which further irritates the oil glands, and a vicious cycle is created.

Blepharitis is the single most common medical eye problem for which people see an ophthalmologist.

We have found that the daily use of B+Z non-Alcohol Toner as an eyelid scrub can prevent recurrent blepharitis.

Blepharitis is a chronic condition that may be very difficult to clear up. It can be one of two types, or a combination.

TYPES OF BLEPHARITIS

- **SEBORRHEIC**—may be associated with dandruff of the scalp or eyebrows
- **STAPHYLOCOCCAL**—a low-grade infection may flare up from time to time in the glands

Symptoms of Blepharitis

People who have blepharitis may experience eye irritation, redness, tearing, feeling of something in the eye, itching, burning, occasional sharp pains, ache in or around the eye, sensitivity to light, blurring, "film" over the eye, crusting or mattering at the base of the eyelashes, and frequent sties or chalazions. The symptoms may be most noticeable upon awakening, because the eyes have been bathing in the irritating secretions of the oil glands all night. During the day, these secretions are partially washed away by the blinking of the eyelids and the flow of tears.

Some of the symptoms of blepharitis may also be caused by other eye problems, such as dry eye syndrome or allergic problems. Many people actually have both dry eye syndrome and blepharitis at the same time.

Causes of Blepharitis

Blepharitis occurs most often in people who have oily skin. People with diabetes and rosacea may also have a slightly higher risk of developing the problem.

Treatments for Blepharitis

A warm, moist washcloth is held against the closed eyelids, rewetting the washcloth with warm water every thirty seconds or so to keep it warm enough. Mild baby shampoo that has been diluted about 50 percent with warm water is applied using a Q-tip to gently scrub the eyelid margins clean by wiping back and forth along the base of the eyelashes on the upper and lower lids. After completing a lid scrub, rinse the eyelids gently with warm water. We have found that using round cosmetic pads moistened first with B+Z Non-Alcohol Toner and later with B+Z Gentle Cleanser are very effective in cleaning the eyelashes and controlling blepharitis. In some cases, a sulfa or antibiotic eye ointment is applied very sparingly along the margin of the lower eyelids. Over-the-counter artificial tear drops can also relieve irritation. The best drops for this purpose are preservative free, which come in tiny single-use plastic containers. The preservatives in regular artificial tear drops can irritate the eye if used too frequently. Exceptionally soothing are homeopathic eye drops (Optique® by Boiron). Although blepharitis is often a chronic, recurring condition, you can usually control the symptoms by keeping up with the lid hygiene routine.

Other Cosmetic Problems of Eyelid Skin

Eyelid dermatitis can appear on the upper eyelids, as well as underneath the lower eye lashes. Usually red, flakey, and swollen in appearance, it can be very uncomfortable. It can be related to products you are using, touching your eyes after touching papers, having manicures with allergenic nail polishes, some prescription drugs, or hair dyes.

For fine eyelid milia, moles, and clogged pores, we use our scarless mole removal technique—a fine wire radiowave electrode (Ellman Surgitron) that can shave off a lump or a bump without leaving a scar.

Xanthalasmas are skin growth lesions that are much larger and deeper than milia, but they are much flatter and have a yellowish tone. Xanthalasmas are sometimes indicative of other disorders, especially elevated cholesterol levels. They often involve orbicularis muscle under the skin as well as the skin.

PTOSIS

Ptosis (pronounced "tosis") is the term applied to a truly droopy eyelid. Some infants are born with ptosis of an eyelid, but for most people, it is something acquired during life. Congenital ptosis should be repaired before the child is five-years-old to avoid the development of a lazy eye with poor vision. Severe ptosis may interfere with peripheral vision, especially the upper half of one's field of vision. Occasionally, the drooping eyelid may even change the curvature of the upper part of the cornea, give you astigmatism, and cause blurring of vision.

Causes of Ptosis

The development of ptosis may indicate a nerve problem that may be a result of serious conditions in the brain, such as tumors, strokes, and aneurysms, or by injuries, diabetes, and migraines. Ptosis may also be secondary to a muscle or nerve condition. For instance, an uncommon cause of ptosis is myasthenia gravis, a muscle disease that causes weakness and sometimes involves only the muscles around the eyes. In older people, ptosis is often caused by a weakening of the levator aponeurosis, a tendonlike sheet that connects the levator muscle to the structures of the eyelid. This is a mechanical problem; the muscle moves normally, but it is out of position and does not lift the eyelid enough.

Surgery for Ptosis

In most cases, the levator muscle can be strengthened or repositioned. In severe cases when the levator muscle is hardly functioning (severe congenital ptosis or ptosis after a stroke where there is loss of nerve function), a sling proce- dure is performed with a special nylon suture, and using it to suspend the upper eyelid from the muscle of the forehead.

To decide which procedure will be best for you, we measure the height of the palpebral fissure (the distance between the edge of the upper lid and the edge of the lower lid) and the distance traveled by the edge of the upper lid as you look up and look down. This measurement determines how well the levator muscle is functioning and what type of surgery is appropriate. When the ptosis may be affecting vision, we perform a visual field test to see how much of the upper field of vision is being blocked by the droopy eyelid.

We can tell if the eyelid lifting muscle (the levator apo- neursis) is out of position because the eyelid looks different. The horizontal crease in the upper eyelid is less prominent, moves higher on the lid, or disappears or the area under the eyebrow appears deep.

This muscle can be corrected with a simple technique of

suturing the aponeurosis back into its correct position. This can be conveniently done during blepharoplasty.

Droopy Eyelid Skin or Dermatochalasis

Droopy eyelids basically fall into one of two categories: dermatochalasis or ptosis.

Dermatochalasis is the presence of excessive and redundant eyelid skin that obscures the upper eyelid lashes and appears to narrow the vertical eye opening and progresses with aging. It is treated with a removal of the excessive skin and laser melting of extra fatty tissue. A true ptosis (muscle out of position) may also be present and should also be repaired at the same time.

ECTROPION

Ectropion is a condition in which the margin of the eyelid turns outward away from the globe. Most cases involve the lower lids. Effects of ectropion include corneal exposure, tearing, keratinization of the conjunctiva inside of the eyelid, and blurring of vision.

Ectropion typically occurs with age, and the lower lid and supportive tendons tends to elongate and become lax. When the margin of the lower eyelid does not touch the eye, the tears do not make it into the tear drainage openings. Tears collect between the eyeball and the lower lid and can cause tears to overflow or irritation. Constant rubbing of the eyes can make it worse. If an ectropion is not corrected, the skin of the eyelid can shrink, and a skin graft may be necessary to correct it.

Correcting Ectropion

If the cornea is significantly exposed from the ectropion, lubrication and moisture shields are helpful. In some cases, taping the lateral canthal skin provides temporary relief. Before surgery, using a lubricating ointment for several days or weeks can help with a keratinized conjunctiva. To avoid worsening the ectropion, always wipe the eyelids in an inward and upward direction.

The basic premise of surgical techniques to treat ectropion is to tighten the lower lid margin and lateral canthal tendon and to rotate the lid margin back into position. An entire segment of the lid on the side away from the nose may be removed to tighten the lid margin. In some cases, the ectropion is very mild but is causing tearing because the opening to the tear drainage system has fallen away from the eye. To treat this condition, the punctum on the lid margin near the nose is rotated into proper position against the eye. Rotating the lid margin inward allows tears to drain away from the eye more normally.

We find a lateral canthal tightening approach to be less invasive. The lateral tarsal strip or canthal application approaches are the most common variations of lateral canthal tightening. These procedures can be performed under local anesthesia and have only four to five days of downtime when performed with the laser as a cutting implement.

ENTROPION

Ectropion and entropion are the different end results of lower lid margin laxity. Either the lashes turn out—ectropion—or in towards the eye—entropion. Often a result of aging, entropion involves an inward turning of the eyelid margin, mostly seen with the lower lids. With entropion, the eyes become irritated by the scraping of the eyelashes against the eyeball. As a result, a muscle imbalance occurs in the eyelid that allows the lid to turn in against the eye and irritate it. Like an old piece of cloth, the lid, as a result of wear and tear, has become stretched and thinned out. Inflammation or irritation of the eye can also coincide with an entropion. Ectropion can also be caused by scarring from injuries, burns, or infection.

A stitch everting the eyelid margin can temporarily lessen the effects of entropion. Lubricants, drops, and protective contact lenses can protect the surface of the eye. Small amounts of botulinum toxin can be used to relax a spastic entropion by weakening the pretarsal orbicularis oculi muscle that pushes the eyelashes against the eye

Surgical procedures to treat entropion involve correcting lower laxity and rotating the lid margin away from the eye. Effective for mild cases, a triangular wedge of tissue is removed from the inside of the lower lid. To correct the horizontal elongation of the lid that occurs with aging, an entire segment of the eyelid may be excised to shorten it. Another approach that restores the eyelid to its original position is done by relocating and repairing the lower lid retractor muscle. Our preferred approach is to use a CO_2 laser to tighten the lateral canthal tendon, and a series of self-dissolving sutures to turn out the eyelashes. This is performed under local anesthesia requiring only several days' downtime.

A combination antibiotic and steroid ointment is placed on sutures after surgery. To relieve swelling, cold compress are applied every fifteen minutes during waking hours. The sutures dissolve after five to seven days. Complications are rare and may include bleeding, swelling, infection, pain, and inadequate reorientation of the lashes. When the CO_2 laser is used there is usually no bruising at all.

EYELID RETRACTION

Eyelid retraction is the term for eyelids that open too widely and produce a wide stare, limiting the ability of the eye to close, exposing the cornea, and causing drying of the cornea. Thyroid eye disease or Grave's disease, is the most common cause of eyelid retraction. It is related to the pull of overactive eyelid muscles; corrective techniques are directed at lessening their pull. Eyelid function, appearance, and comfort can be improved by surgery that weakens the muscles that open the eye.

Injecting botulinum toxin into the inside lining of the upper lid onto the levator and Müller's muscles is one method to treat upper eyelid retraction that is associated with thyroid eye disease. After lid retraction surgery, botulinum toxin can be used to relax the eyelid opening muscles, allowing them to heal more effectively in their new position.

In some cases, what appears to be a drooping upper eyelid is actually a retracted opposite upper eyelid. The "droopy" eyelid is only droopy in comparison to the opposite lid, which is actually retracted superiorly. The lid retraction may be partially hidden by excess skin and only becomes apparent if the lid skin is gently lifted.

Lower eyelid retraction, like lower lid ectropion, can be caused by a compromised support system but also by the shrinkage of any of several tissue layers, including skin, muscle, and retractors. This combination of horizontal laxity and vertical shortening causes the lower lid to pull downward or retract below the cornea, and as a result, exposing the white of the eye.

Lid retraction can occur naturally with aging and laxity of the supporting eyelid tendons, with overactive thyroid disease, or when too much eyelid skin has been removed during surgery.

There is no one all-inclusive approach to the correction of lower eyelid retraction. Most cases can be corrected; all can be improved.

Each case must be individually analyzed and a customized surgical plan offered.

LOWER EYELID RETRACTION TECHNIQUES

- Support System Reinforcement (Canthoplasty)
- Grafting of an Internal Spacer (Upper lid tarsus and conjunctiva, Ear Cartilage, Hard Palate).
- Skin Grafting
- Midface or Thread Lifts
- Augmentation Of Insufficient Bony Support Below The Eye

LAGOPHTHALMOS—INABILITY TO CLOSE COMPLETELY

The upper eyelid is responsible for 75 percent of eyelid closure, while the lower eyelid has a less significant role.

Lagophthalmos can be the result of facial paralysis (Bell's palsy, stroke, tumor) or can be caused by mechanical limitation of eyelid closure (scarring from accident or previous surgery). Each surgery performed on the delicate eyelid inevitably causes some scarring and may reduce the casual blink, forced voluntary closure of the eyelids, or result in lagophthalmos.

CAUSES OF LAGOPHTHALMOS

- An impairment of mechanical closure of the lids (too much skin removed during surgery, accidents, burns)
- Bacterial infection
- Bell's palsy
- Cerebral vascular accidents (strokes)
- Exophthalmos (the eye itself is pushed too far forward so that the eyelids cannot close over the eye which occurs with overactive thyroid conditions or tumors behind the eye)
- Neurosurgical procedures
- Paralysis of orbicularis oculi (stroke, tumors, or too much botulinum toxin)
- Trauma

Because the eyelids protect and nourish our eyes, the loss of blinking or eyelid closure can risk the health of your eyes.

POSSIBLE COMPLICATIONS OF LAGOPHTHALMOS

- Severe dry eye and discomfort—drying of the cornea
- Corneal keratitis (inflammation of the cornea)
- Corneal erosion (similar to a corneal abrasion)
- Corneal ulceration (infection of the cornea)
- Decrease or loss of vision because of corneal scarring

With older blepharoplasty techniques, temporary lagophthalmos often occurred that was more apparent during sleep, when there is only gentle eyelid closure. Lagophthalmos can persist for weeks after surgery, and the lower eyelid may be massaged upward to lubricate the lower cornea. This area is affected the most by the upper eyelid's inability to close completely. Eye drops and ointments may be used throughout the day to help maintain a well lubricated eye. Fortunately, our blepharoplasty patients no longer have to suffer with this post-operative discomfort.

By removing less upper eyelid skin, not removing ANY lower eyelid skin, and tightening the appropriate supportive eyelid tendons, lagophthalmos following blepharoplasty can be <u>completely</u> avoided.

Lagophthalmos that is caused by excessive skin removal or internal scarring can be a serious problem that compromises the health of the eye surface. For severe cases, surgery may be necessary to remove scarring and to replace tissue. A graft of the inside lining of the upper lid can be used to build up the inner lining of the lower eyelid. In extreme cases skin grafts taken from the skin behind the ear (this has the closest color and texture match) are placed into the upper or lower eyelids. Usually a lateral canthoplasty will be performed at the same time to give additional support and elevation to the lower lid.

CHAPTER 7

Eye Enhancement—Artistry in Micropigmentation & Lashes

The eyebrows and eyelashes frame the eyes, and aging causes them to thin and fade and lose definition.

Re-establishing structural definition to the eyelid area is a critical step in aesthetic facial rejuvenation. As the hair thins and the colors fade, the eyes lack presence, making the face monochromatic. Artistic micropigmentation techniques can add the finishing touch to a facial rejuvenating program.

Regardless of your skin type the final touch after your blepharoplasty will be the enhancement of your eyelashes. Are they full enough? Do they accent your eyes enough? Are you missing eyelashes? Have recurrent bouts of blepharitis caused your lashes to fall out? Have you have small growths removed from your eyelids causing loss of lashes?

This is when micropigmentation of your eyelashes can really enhance your appearance. This technique does not replace make-up, it is only used to make your eyelashes appear more luxuriant and full—and it will stay in place for years! For an extra three dimensional effect we can actually also add hair, one hair at a time. The individual hairs are taken from your scalp.

What is micropigmentation?

Micropigmentation is similar to tattooing. It can be used to mimic eyeliner, eyebrow pencil, lip liner, and lipstick. When performed artistically, semi-permanent make-up can appear entirely natural. We often use our technique to camouflage tattooing that has given the eyebrow an inappropriate arch or color. To keep it looking fresh, we recommend touch-ups yearly. The technique of micropigmentation involves metabolically inert pigment granules implanted below the epidermis for cosmetic and/or corrective enhancement. Micropigmentation is used to enhance facial features—eyebrows, lashes, and lips—and to improve discolored scars and vitiligo (uneven loss of pigmentation).

Women are motivated to have micropigmentation when they are active in sports, allergic to ingredients in make-up, have difficulty applying make-up because of poor vision or arthritis, or have thinning eyebrows.

Our micropigmentation technique is very gentle and the procedure is individualized for each patient. The colors are customized so that you can choose which tone and shade suit you best. The brow shape is designed to accentuate your eyes and to enhance your facial features. We use a computerized, digitalized machine that does not traumatize the skin. The results are longstanding, but need to be touched up each year. This will give you the chance to change the color and shape slightly if you like.

WHERE CAN MICROPIGMENTATION BE DONE?	
• Eyeliner	• Lip color
• Brows	• Repigmenting scars
• Lip line	• Nipple reconstruction

If you are considering micropigmentation to enhance your eyeliner, eyebrow, or lip pigmentation, we will examine your eyes and eyelids and give you an overall facial analysis. We will pencil in one side of your face so that you can observe the proposed changes before and after the procedure.

How is micropigmentation performed?

We will use a tattoo pen to inject semi-permanent, sterile ink into your skin in a series of dots. Each procedure takes about thirty to sixty minutes. Topical numbing cream and local anesthetic are used to make the procedure comfortable. All coloring may initially appear brighter or darker than desired, but will fade to the desired color over several days. Some of the tattooed areas may appear crusty for a few days. It is important that you keep these areas well lubricated and do not pick off the crusts to avoid losing pigment. You may also have some swelling for two to five days.

The procedure is relatively quick; an upper and lower lash line takes about thirty to forty minutes. There is local swelling and minimal discomfort following tattooing. The treated area usually looks normal within a week to ten days. You will use an antibiotic ointment following the procedure four times daily for one week. Results can be seen immediately although the final end result will be seen in about three weeks.

How do we choose the pigments?

Human skin color is the result of the various combinations of three pigment colors: brown-black (melanin), yellow (phaeomelanin, indole, carotene, xanthophylls), and red (hemoglobins and dopachrome). We will evaluate your natural skin pigment and mix the appropriate combination of colors that suite you best and that you find pleasing. The pigments used are made from safe, non-reactive compounds approved by the FDA. The dyes are available in many colors and can be matched to skin tones for customized results.

The universally accepted foundation for all color theories is the cool/warm concept. Skin will show either a blue (blue-pink) undertone or a yellow (golden-beige) undertone. We determine the skin undertone before proceeding with the integration of additional colors. This is important, because the colors that we choose will look different in the bottle than they do on your skin. We use a pointillism principle of optical mixture on a microlevel of depositing isolated colors until a natural blend is achieved. We also blend the dyes before implanting them. We are not camouflaging the natural skin undertone, but rather utilizing the skin undertone as a canvas to integrate complementary hues.

Semi-Permanent Eyeliner

Eyeliner can be applied in many styles and colors, from soft, natural-looking lash enhancement to a defined line. For semi-permanent eyeliner, the shade should match the natural eyelash color as close as possible. This gives a very natural look that can be covered by other colors if you choose to wear a darker color. For pale blondes or fair skinned women, we generally do not choose black, which may look ashy. Enhanced eyes will have a darker, thicker, lash line. A micro needle is used to achieve a thinly lined look.

How is the pigment placed?

The pigment is placed on the eyelid in a series of dots. The end effect is that of an eyeliner or eyelash enhancement. Most often, the pigment will be placed along the lower lid lashes at their bases. A small area is left unpigmented to avoid the impression of closing the lids with the upper and the lower pigment lines meeting. The artistic flavor of the procedure is gained by placing more or less pigment in three segments of the line. If you use eyeliner on your lid margins, you should be aware that permanent eyeliner will not resemble your usual makeup technique because the micropigmentation technique is much more delicate and exact than a pencil.

In general, the upper eyelid pigment line is thicker and longer than the lower lid line because there are more lashes on the upper lid and it is longer than the lower lid. By leaving the most inferior row of the upper eyelid eyelashes unpigmented, we can create a more open appearance to the eye. In most women, the segment closest to the nose on the upper and lower lids should have thin lines, with only the starting point, not the thickness varying.

As the line moves away from the nose, the amount and placement of pigment can vary. A flaring and lift can be accomplished by placing more pigment. The increase in the pigment in this zone tends to enlarge eyes and bring them forward. The variability of the temporal zone allows the practitioner to modify the thickness of the line as well as the line's endpoint. The more flaring created by the disposition of the pigment, the wider and more prominent the eye will appear. The endpoint of the line can affect the optical illusion of separation within a certain zone. The temporal zone next to the lateral canthus and a corresponding upper and lower eyelid are considered the shift zone areas. The perceived appearance of wide or close separation of the eyes is affected by pigmentation in this area. The middle or central zone functions as a blending zone between the nasal and temporal area. In this zone, many subtle aspects of artistic optical illusions can be performed by altering the shape, affecting size, and enhancing set by the placement of the pigment.

Eye Shape

The shape of an eye is determined by the arch of the upper and lower lid contours, the palpebral fissure, and the relationship of the medial and lateral canthal attachments. We modify our application technique for each eye shape.

Angular Eyes

In eyes that have an angular appearance, the lid contour can be softened by adding additional pigment in the superior temporal zone of the upper eyelid with an extra row of dots that will give a more rounded appearance to the eyes.

Round Eyes

By adding extra pigment in the temporal zone of the upper and lower lid, the round eyes are made more prominent and accentuated. By using thinner lines a round eye may be given more of an almond shape when the pigment line is extended nasally using the roll technique.

Almond Eyes

In eyes that have the ideal almond appearance, it is best to just follow the actual lid contours and avoid excessive pigmentation. A small amount extra pigment temporally can give more prominence to the eye.

Asian Eyes

It is important to ask the patient whether cosmetic surgery of the epicanthal fold or lid crease is contemplated in the future. If eyelid surgery is planned, we recommend deferring the blepharopigmentation until further surgery has been completed. We can achieve a subtle lifting effect by adding more pigment to the temporal zone of the upper lid. The epicanthal fold can be deemphasized with the placement of a thin delicate line in the nasal zone of the upper lid.

EYEBROWS

The eyebrows are the most popular area for micropigmentation.

From providing a basic guideline for you to follow to pencil them yourself, to total brow recreation, micropigmented brows can range from a few hair strokes to dramatic, fully colored brows. Sometimes we use the individual hair-like strokes technique, which may look very natural if the pigment is a soft, light color. Two to three colors are often used in a single application to simulate natural eyebrows. We consider your hair color and skin tones to select the ideal pigment for you. When selecting an eyebrow shape, we avoid trends or unrealistic super high arches and a dated look because micropigmentation can last years.

Typically for the eyebrows, two treatments are needed and should be spaced at least one or more weeks apart. Our digitalized micropigmentation needles are set to penetrate the skin at a specific depth of one to two millimeters. Patients can resume normal activities within twenty-four hours.

LIP COLOR AND SHAPE

As lip pigmentation fades, the lips lose definition and appear smaller. This accentuates the fact that lips do lose volume with aging. Lip shape, definition, volume, and position can be rejuvenated with a combined technique of Perlane® and Restylane® volume augmentation, mouth corner elevation with botulinum toxin and fillers (Perlane® or Sculptra®), and micropigmentation. Sufficient anesthesia is achieved with topical Photocaine cream.

By redefining the lip pigment, less fillers will need to be used to maintain lip volume.

Are there any risks?

The greatest risk with micropigmentation is having an untrained individual or someone who does not share your aesthetic outlook perform this procedure.

If you have a history of cold sores we will start you on Acyclovir one day before your micropigmentation is performed. Infection or irritation can be caused by contaminated needles, non-medical grade ink. If your micropigmented-eyebrow is placed high, you will have a permanent look of surprise. Because of the precision involved, especially around the eyes, removal can be difficult as lasers can damage the hair follicles and result in loss of eyelashes or eyebrows.

- This is a semi-permanent procedure; laser surgery is required to remove pigment.
- Avoid direct sunlight, do not apply make-up or wear contact lenses for a few days
- Avoid swimming or getting the area wet for a week.
- Allergic reactions and infections are rare.

- Certain pigments may cause interference with cranial MRI scans.

- Needles inserted too deeply in the skin can cause bleeding, spreading of pigments, scarring, and damage to hair follicles.

EYELASH RESTORATION

Assessing the thickness, density, color, and contour of the eyebrows and eyelashes is essential in evaluation of periorbital rejuvenation. To create the frame for the eyes we direct our attention to eyebrow and eyelash enhancement. For maximum effect and benefit, we plan for eyebrow and eyelash rejuvenation when a blepharoplasty is being planned.

Eyelash transplant surgery is performed to add eyelashes to the upper eyelid. Transplantation is the only procedure used to restore eyelash hair. To perform eyelash transplantation, we obtain a graft of hair from the back of the scalp, where the hair is the thickest. The graft is divided into single-hair follicular units, and any excess fat, dermis, and epidermis are trimmed in order to make each graft very fine; excess tissue around the hair can compromise the survival of the graft. After anesthetizing the eyelid and protecting the cornea with an eye shield, we use a very fine transplanting needle to implant about twenty to thirty hairs into the eyelids. Each hair is implanted one at a time. The procedure takes about an hour. After transplantation, the new lashes grow longer than natural lashes and therefore must be trimmed regularly.

Itching is a common and troublesome post-operative problem. If you give in to temptation and scratch, there is risk for dislodging the hair grafts or initiating infection. Eyeglasses can be worn to deter you from scratching. The transplanted hairs can be trained in the direction of the other eyelashes with lash oil and an eyelash curler.

Eyebrow Reconstruction

You may want us to correct defects in your eyebrow caused by trauma, burns, or surgery. Many of our patients requesting eyebrow transplantation want to fill out patchy eyebrows. This can be done with single follicular unit hair transplantation or sometimes removing the scar and reconstructing the area with tissue flaps.

A strip of hair-bearing skin and subcutaneous tissue is removed from a donor area on the scalp and grafted into the surgically-prepared eyebrow site. Transplants can also camouflage scars in the eyebrow area. The transplant procedure is performed by selecting a hair-bearing area of scalp with hair that is of appropriate texture and orientation to serve as eyebrow hair. Micrografts of one to two hairs placed into incisions should be used for eyebrow reconstruction. The graft sites are marked with indelible pen. As with eyelash transplant surgery, local anesthesia is administered and a hair graft is then taken. This graft is divided into single hair grafts, which are then implanted one by one. Eyebrows may require six hundred single-hair grafts, and the procedure may take several hours, depending on the extent of the reconstruction.

With careful attention to the direction and angle of the eyebrow hairs' growth, we can transform patchy or absent eyebrows into natural-looking eyebrows.

We have found that about 90 percent of newly transplanted hairs survive and create dense, full eyebrows.

Transplantation to Correct Eyebrow Loss

Transplantation of hair to the eyebrow can recreate the eyebrow in a natural contour. We work closely with our patients to outline the eyebrow area to conform to the natural symmetry of your face. Depending on the size of the area to be transplanted, more than one transplant session may be required; two or more sessions several months apart are common.

Donor hair for the transplant is taken from a site that furnishes finer rather than coarser hair; finer hair is a better "match" for eyebrow hair. Donor hair is transplanted as micrografts of one to two hairs. Each graft is placed into an incision prepared for it. The use of single hairs or micrografts permits meticulous adherence to the eyebrow contour for a natural appearance. As the transplanted hairs grow in their new position they may require occasional trimming as well as "training" with gel or wax.

Results of Eyebrow and Eyelash Transplantation

Both eyelash and eyebrow transplantations have very few complications. There is no visible scarring or tufting, and the results appear quite natural. There may be some bleeding, minor pain, and swelling. Eyebrows and eyelashes make an important contribution to facial symmetry and presentation of yourself to others.

EYEBROWS & EYELASHES MAY BE LOST IN MANY WAYS

- Physical trauma—accident or thermal, chemical, or electrical burns

- Systemic or local disease that causes loss of eyebrows and/or eyelashes

- Congenital inability to grow eyebrows and/or eyelashes

- Plucking to reshape the eyebrow that results in permanent loss

- Self-inflicted obsessive plucking of eyebrows and/or eyelashes (trichotillomania)

- Medical or surgical treatments that result in loss— radiation therapy, chemotherapy, surgical removal of tumor

Before transplantation or surgical restoration, your health must be in good condition and the underlying causes of the hair loss must be under control to make sure the procedure is successful. In cases that involve trauma, burns, or surgery that may have formed scar tissue, reconstructive surgery may be necessary before eyebrow and/or eyelash restoration. The degree of eyebrow loss can vary from partial to complete; the degree of loss will be a consideration in the selection of the restoration procedure.

CHAPTER 8

Tender
Loving Care
For the Eyes

Taking good care of the eyelid area before and after surgery will lead to superior results, and prolong the benefits.

How to Prepare for Eyelid Surgery

There are many things that you can do to prepare for your surgery that will minimize your chances of bleeding during surgery or bruising after your surgery. Simply stopping all anti-inflammatory pills or capsules and vitamin E will help. Taking Arnica Montana, Papain, and Bromelain will also decrease bruising and accelerate healing. Vitamin C, Alpha Lipoic Acid and zinc will increase protein synthesis and promote more rapid and stronger healing. Anti-oxidants—green tea, grapeseed, blueberry, lavender, ginger, and Coenzyme Q10- will scavenge free radicals and promote faster healing. Lymphatic drainage massage will open up the lymphatic drainage channels and allow more rapid diminution of swelling following non-invasive and surgical procedures.

BZ PREOP INSTRUCTIONS

* Stop all products containing aspirin two weeks before surgery

* Increase intake of vitamin C to at least 3,000 mg a day (1,000 mg after each meal) beginning two weeks before surgery

* Begin taking the following two weeks before surgery:

Co Q-10	10 mg
Alpha-Lipoic Acid	100mg
L-Carnosine	25 mg
Flax Seed Powder	100mg
Magnesium Sterate	5mg
Zinc Oxide	15mg
Lavender	15mg

- Begin taking sublingual Arnica Montana pellets (strength C6, five pellets sublingual four times daily) two days before surgery

- Begin taking Bromalein, Papain, green tea, ginger, and blueberry capsules the day before surgery

- Begin lymphatic drainage massage one day before surgery

HELPING YOUR EYELIDS HEAL

In order to assist with a speedy healing process, we have developed formulas for natural healing aids to reduce bruising and swelling after surgery.

B+Z DAILY SUPPLEMENT

Contains these important vitamins and nutrients:

Vitamin E	30 OU
Co Q-10	10 mg
Alpha-Lipoic Acid	100 mg
L-Carnosine	25 mg
Flax Seed Powder	100 mg
Magnesium Sterate	5 mg
Zinc Oxide	15mg
Lavender	15mg

B+Z HEALING SUPPLEMENT
Contains 1000mg of vitamin C and bromelain, papain, green tea, ginger, blueberry, grapeseed extract.

POST-OP INSTRUCTIONS

- Continue lymphatic drainage massage daily for five days if possible.

- Cool compresses for at least 15 minutes every hour for the first 36 hours.

- Apply ophthalmic antibiotic ointment to eyelids twice daily for one week.

- Apply copper peptide cream to resurfaced eyelids four times daily for one week.

- Continue Arnica Montana for five days.

- Continue vitamin C, Bromelain, Papain and green tea, ginger, lavender for at least two weeks.

- After surgery, apply ice or cold compresses to the eyelids. Blood-tinged (pink) discharge may occur and this is normal.

Because the eyelids are extremely vascular, they heal rapidly with minimal risk of infection. It is common to experience some mild bruising and discoloration around the eye. This is minimized when the carbon dioxide laser is used as an incisional tool—blood vessels are sealed as the surgery is performed.

RECOVERY TIPS

- Apply antibiotic ophthalmic ointment at bedtime for one week.

- For the first 48 hours after surgery, apply bags of frozen peas with a piece of sterile gauze between the eyelid and the peas for 10 to 15 minutes every hour while awake. After the first 48 hours, repeat four times a day for the next two days.

- While some discharge is not unusual after laser resurfacing of the eyelids, severe discomfort is unusual.

- Do not rub your eyes. To avoid infection, wash your hands before and after administering any medications.

- Moisten eyelids in the morning with sterile gauze soaked in sterile saline solution to separate the eyelids if they stick together.

- Use one antibiotic drop with mild steroid in each eye two times a day for one week after surgery. Do not pull on your eyelids. Lay back, with your eyes closed, put two drops on the inside corner of your eye, near the nose, then open your eyes. The drops will go into your eyes.

- You will have lower eyelid dressings after resurfacing (this will allow you to heal faster), you may shower but do not wet your head or allow water onto the dressings until after your first post-op visit, when the dressings will be removed.

- After the lower lid dressings have been removed, your eyes can get wet, but pat them dry gently.

- You can resume taking aspirin one week after surgery if no bleeding occurs. You may continue all other medications, including any glaucoma medications.

Swelling typically is visible the morning after surgery and increases over the next thirty-six hours. By the third post-op day it begins to decrease dramatically. Swelling is always worse in the morning but dissipates with the effects of gravity after being up and about during the day. To decrease swelling and the risk of postoperative bleeding, keep your heart above your head when lying down. Sleep on two pillows. Lymphatic drainage massage and Arnica Montana will also help.

During the first forty-eight hours after surgery, your vision will be blurry from the swelling and the antibiotic ointment. It is not uncommon to see swelling in the upper eyelids, lower eyelids, the cheek, and lower facial area during the two to three days following the surgery. Since the advent of our laser techniques, bruising is less common, and is usually minimal. The coloring of bruising goes from red to blue, blue to brown, and finally brown to yellow. The blood breakdown products are gradually absorbed by blood vessels and the lymphatic drainage of the face. Infection is also extremely rare and laser technique makes it even less common. The discoloration of bruising is different from the redness, pain, and swelling of the tissues due to infection.

During the days following the surgery this swelling will move lower on the face. You may even notice it on your cheeks and jowls. After laser resurfacing, we will apply an adhesive dressing to your lower eyelids and leave it in place for the first week. Because your upper eyelids have to open and close, we cannot apply a dressing to the upper lids. They will ooze slightly and be red on the first day and then become dry and crusty for the remaining seven days following the surgery. Ophthalmic antibiotic ointment must be applied to the upper eyelid skin every four hours for the first week after surgery.

Sometimes the eye itself can appear to be bloodshot. This is not unusual and can last several days.

Tearing is common and can be controlled by frequent, complete blinking and topical artificial tears such as Refresh eye drops. All topical tears are available over-the-counter. Burning, tearing, and even foreign-body sensation can occur because of incomplete blinking (from the swelling) and drying. Some of our patients experience numbness of their upper lids following upper eyelid surgery. This will diminish over several months.

The redness and swelling begins to disappear on the third post-op day and should significantly dissipate one week after surgery. Warm compresses and Arnica Montana can be used as long as bruising is present and swelling persists. These compresses promote healing by increasing the blood supply to the injured area. Swelling is always worse in the morning but improves during the day as gravity moves the built up fluid from the eyelids to the lower face. To reduce eyelid swelling, elevate the head by sleeping with extra pillows.

Makeup may be used seven days after the procedure.

SPECIALIST SKINCARE

We have embraced aestheticians and exchanged learning experiences since the First Annual Eyelid Rejuvenation Symposium that we hosted in the mid-1980's. At that landmark conference our podium was filled with a distinguished faculty of aestheticians, surgeons, dermatologists, and scientists. And so began our long and productive relationship. The ideal of aestheticians working alongside physicians is now at hand. More and more physicians and surgeons are finally understanding the insights, and appreciating the contributions of aestheticians.

The delicate and thin eyelid tissue demands cautious care. Constant exposure to the sun without the protection of sunglasses, sun block, and anti-oxidants will have a direct effect on the breakdown of the skin over a period of time, weakening the elastin and collagen fibers. The eyelids are also one of the most common areas on the face for skin cancers. Any new growths or crusting areas must be examined and biopsied.

Allergies and skin sensitivity around the eyelids are not unusual. More than fifty percent of women complain of sensitive eyes, feelings of discomfort, localized mild pain, dryness, mild redness, a feeling of heavy lids, and tearing. Because of the high sensitivity of the eye contour area and the defense mechanisms within, it is essential that all products you use on your eyes are effective, safe, and irritation-free. Repeated allergic reactions can stretch the eyelid skin creating a loose, crepey texture.

The skin's semi-permeable barrier is particularly vulnerable in the eye contour area, which allows any substance applied to the skin to penetrate it more easily than elsewhere in the body. This delicate area requires a specialized skincare regimen for protection and repair. Eye moisturizers have to be nourishing, yet more delicate than facial moisturizers. Anti-oxidants must be potent but less irritating.

These factors have led us to the exciting development of an advanced product—Beautif-Eye™ that is a unique combination of Brazilian rain forest anti-oxidants, collagen stimulators, lightening agents, wrinkle relaxers, and rich moisturizers developed for the specific requirements of eyelid skin. To restore and normalize this barrier, we have included Cupuacu butter and Andiroba oil. These substances strengthen the eye contour and hydrate the skin. It also contains the anti-oxidants vitamins C and E to protect the delicate eyelid skin, and willowherb to calm the skin. This is a perfect product for the eye that incorporates leading technologies clinically proven to improve wrinkles, lines, and dark areas around the eye. It also uses special emollients to soothe the skin and provide exceptional moisturizing and softening properties. After application, the first results may be visible within one half hour. Using it every morning and evening can lead to long lasting improvement.

B+Z DAILY EYE CARE REGIMEN

We have designed this treatment to release tension and fatigue around the eye area, to cleanse the lashes, to help improve the hydration and suppleness of the eyelid skin, and to lessen the appearance of fine lines and wrinkles.

MORNING ROUTINE

- Scrub your eyelashes with B+Z non-alcohol toner, removing any morning crusts from your eyes. Yes, men, you too.
- Wash your eyelids and face with B+Z Gentle White Cleanser.
- Apply Beautif-Eye™ Nourishing Cream to your upper and lower lids.
- Apply sun block.
- Wear sunglasses.

EVENING ROUTINE

- Men, scrub your eyelashes with B+Z Non-Alcohol Toner.
- Women, remove your make-up with B+Z Gentle White Cleanser and then B+Z Non-Alcohol Toner.
- For eye relaxation, apply compresses soaked in soothing B+Z Non-Alcohol Toner to your closed eyelids and leave them in place for 5 minutes.
- Gently massage your eyelids and eyebrows
- To complete the treatment, finish with Beautif-Eye™ Nourishing cream

BEAUTIFEYE REGIMEN— CORRECT, PROTECT, RENEW™

- Eye creams are cream based emollients designed to moisturize, hydrate, and improve the suppleness of the skin. Beautifeye sets the standard for a new generation of eye creams with more effective Brazilian rainforest botanical skin barrier enhancers, anti-oxidants, soothing agents, and muscle relaxing polypeptides.

- B+Z Crystal C Gel is ideal for younger patients, used nightly for its anti-oxidant and light moisturizing effects.

- For additional lighten effect, powerful B+Z clarifying lotions can be added to the regimen.

The patient's role is also important in maintaining a rejuvenating effect. Patients can contribute to their skincare in beneficial ways by using home care products, protecting their skin against UV rays, and by quitting smoking and limiting their alcohol intake. We recommend regular follow-up visits to establish treatment goals and facilitate the maintenance of the overall rejuvenating effect. In our practices, we pride ourselves on forming close personal relationships with our patients based on trust, open communication, and continuity of care.

CHAPTER 9

The Beauty of Botulinum Toxin

Botox® represents the single most significant advancement in non-surgical aesthetic medicine of the past decade.

Our initial experience with botulinum was when Dr. Bosniak directed the clinical trials in 1980–1981 at New York's Manhattan Eye, Ear & Throat Hospital for the treatment of uncontrollable eyelid blinking—blepharospasm. That era seems like ancient history now that Botox® has become a household name and, in the last decade, has revolutionized aesthetic medicine.

Botulinum toxin is the most commonly performed cosmetic treatment in the United States. Even though its current FDA cosmetic approval is for the treatment of glabellar furrows, many physicians have been utilizing it off label to treat other areas of the face and neck with dramatic results. Although allergies to Botox® are exceptionally rare, Botox® is not recommended for anyone with an allergy to albumin or who is taking aminoglycoside antibiotics.

The concept of relaxing facial muscles and diminishing their secondary wrinkle-producing effects has become a basic technique in facial rejuvenation. It is a foundation on which other non-invasive and surgical procedures can be built. Botox® can be used by itself to achieve the desired results. We also use it as a component in our menu of combined therapies. These techniques are in a state of evolution as new technologies are introduced and our experience increases.

We instruct our patients that the goal of treatment is not complete immobilization of the facial muscles or a flat, immovable surface. Our therapeutic goal is a natural, relaxed look—to soften and diminish lines and furrows—not necessarily to obliterate them. We have been emphasizing this point since our Keynote Address to the 28th Congress of the Brazilian Ophthalmologic Society in Salvador, Bahia on September 5, 1995.

Horizontal forehead creases respond well to botulinum toxin therapy and usually do not require filling. However, within the one centimeter "no Botox®" zone above the eyebrows, filling works well to supplement softening of the forehead lines. This technique is especially useful in patients where a Botox® brow lift has been performed to raise the level of the eyebrows and to create a more pleasing arch. To avoid flattening an eyebrow arch, we may use fillers to soften forehead lines. Because the position of your eyebrows represent different emotions, it is important to retain normal movement so that you can express these emotions, and to avoid changing your eyebrows to a position that makes you appear tired, angry, or surprised.

"Losing Your 11"

The area between the eyebrows—which we can call the number "11" because of the formation of the creases in that area—is managed well with botulinum toxin when the vertical furrows are apparent only during frowning. However, static furrows that are visible at rest will require fillers as well as muscle relaxation from Botox®. Both treatments can be effectively and efficiently done during one visit. The depressions are filled and then Botox® is used on the muscles that cause furrowing. This combined approach yields more complete and longer-lasting results than when either treatment is used alone. The horizontal crease over the bridge of the nose that is not completely reduced after treatment can also be filled.

Botulinum toxin type A binds where the nerve attaches to the muscle and blocks the chemical that causes the nerve impulses that contract the muscle. This bond is permanent and the chemical release of the nerve endings begins only again when the nerve sprouts a new endplate in three to four months. This means that even if a higher dose of Botox® is given, the results may not necessarily last longer. We aim for just the right dose of Botox®—enough to give the desired effect that lasts as long as possible. The clinical effects after Botox® injections begin after three to five days and the final effects are evident in seven to ten days.

Botulinum Toxin Types

Botox® has become synonymous with botulinum toxin type
A, but Botox® is a specific brand name for a specific product
that has been highly refined and widely tested. We have had
25 years of experience using this product. Our experience
has been primarily with botulinum toxin type A (Botox®,
Allergan), but we have also used botulinum toxin type B
(Myobloc®, Solstice Sciences).

Dr. Zilkha has used Dysport® in Brazil (will become
Reloxan™ in the US) and is currently conducting studies
evaluating the effectiveness of combination therapies using
Botox® and Reloxan™. Dysport® is a type A botulinum
toxin, but its effects are "heavier" than Botox®. Three to five
units of Dysport® are equivalent to one unit of Botox®. At
the current time Dysport® is undergoing clinical trials for
FDA approval in the United States and will be launched as
Reloxin® in the near future. A new botulinum toxin type A
product—Puretox® (Mentor)—is also in development.

We have all heard about illegal botulinum products and
"Chinese Botox®". These products have not undergone the
rigorous clinical and purity trials that the name-branded
products have. These products can be extremely dangerous.
Always make sure that your doctor is using a name brand
botulinum toxin product.

Bethany's Lower Face

We can clearly recall meeting Bethany, a 61-year-old lady who had never tried any rejuvenating procedures before. She had heard about many things, but had never tried any of the non-invasive treatments and of course would not even consider any cosmetic surgical procedures. After reading all the articles that we had written about Botox® and looking at the before and after photos our textbooks, she decided that trying Botox® to relax her crow's feet and the "11" between her eyebrows would not be a bad idea. Bethany was mainly concerned with the obvious wrinkles and furrows between her eyebrows and around her eyes. She came back for her one week follow-up. She could see the improvement and was very pleased, but we decided that a little more Botox® between the eyebrows would enhance the improvement. We were aiming for elimination of the "11", but not complete immobility. She called us a week later and said that she looked terrible, much older than she had before. We asked her to come in to see us right away. As soon as we saw her we were immediately impressed with how great her upper face looked. Her crow's feet and her "11" were gone. Her eyebrows had a pleasant arch. She looked well rested and extremely natural. So what was the problem? Her upper face looked so great that now the shadows and wrinkles of her lower face really bothered her. We used Botox® to relax the muscles that pulled down the corners of her mouth and then Restylane® and Perlane® to soften her naso-labial folds, prop up the corners of her mouth, and fill in her marionette lines. When we freshened up her lower face to match her upper face, she was very happy.

THE PERIORAL AREA

The lower face and perioral area in the past have been off limits to the use of Botox® until we figured out the intricacies of muscle interplay and balance in that area. Botox® in combination with fillers and tissue tightening techniques, has revolutionized treatment of this area, just as Bethany's story above illustrates.

Midface bony atrophy can be non-invasively counteracted with a new intraoral device. Lost dental volume can be replaced. Then the perioral skin can be tightened and plumped. Our **BZ Lift** will tighten jowls and decrease marionette lines after the muscles that pull down the lower face—platysma –and corners of the mouth—depressor angulli oris—have been treated with Botox®. Any remaining folds or grooves are filled with Restylane®, Perlane®, or Sculptra®.

Your upper lip muscle (orbicularis oris) that creates vertical lines can be relaxed with Botox® alone or treated with Botox® and then filled with Restylane® Fine Lines or CosmoDerm® for longer lasting results. These folds are particularly prominent in smokers. Small amounts (one unit) can be used in four spots in the upper and lower lip borders. Botox® has to be placed in exactly the right spot to avoid any mouth asymmetry when you are smiling. Deeper furrows can be removed with ablative lasers (carbon dioxide or erbium), but require about one week of downtime. Laser treatments are much more effective after the lip muscle has been treated with Botox®. Any remaining fine lines can be filled with CosmoDerm®.

You may have never had a full upper lip and now want one. Or you may have had a full upper lip and watched it get thinner and then disappear. Any loss of volume can be replaced with fillers. Loss of the pink lip border can be replaced with our micropigmentation techniques. Botox® will help raise droopy corners of your mouth. The depressor anguli oris is the muscle that pulls down the corners of the mouth. It can be treated with Botox® to slightly raise the corners of the mouth, making Restylane®, Perlane®, Sculptra®, or Radiesse™ more effective when filling marionette lines.

We will discuss all of these techniques in greater detail in Chapter 13 on perioral rejuvenation.

FACIAL ANATOMY

A thorough and intimate knowledge of facial anatomy is a prerequisite for understanding how to effectively use Botox®. This understanding will allow the creative, effective, and safe use of botulinum toxin.

Using the Right Dosage

The goal of botulinum toxin therapy is to use the smallest dosage that produces an optimal effect. This will allow continued use of Botox® for years without any lessening of the effects. In fact, most patients may require even lower doses of Botox® after receiving treatments for several years.

Patients often say that the botulinum toxin given to them by another doctor did not work. It is not that the Botox® did not work—they were not given a sufficient dose or they needed Botox® and filler in combination. Using an adequate dosage for each muscle group is the key. In some facial areas—like "your 11" or marionette lines—a combination of Botox® and fillers will be needed to attain an adequate result.

With botulinum toxin, an insufficient dose will yield an insufficient result.

Botulinum toxin is delivered as a freeze dried powder in a glass jar. It has to be diluted before it can be used. Depending on which muscles need to be treated, we will dilute it to an appropriate strength. If it is diluted too much, it will result in a less effective treatment that does not last as long. By the same token, we avoid making the dilution too strong as this can result in a less than ideal cosmetic outcome. We can always add more if you need it. Since you will not see the full effect for seven to ten days, we request that you come back for a dose adjustment in one to two weeks following your initial treatment session.

PRE BOTOX® PROTOCOL

We take great care to avoid any bruising during your Botox® treatment. If a patient gets a bruise, they are usually very unhappy with their injector. We also take our time to do the treatment; it should not be rushed. We want our patients to have a pleasant experience during their treatment and to leave without any evidence that they have had anything done. To avoid bruising and to decrease the possibility of any downtime, we have our patients follow a tried and true recovery regimen.

Begin taking five Arnica Montana C 6 pellets four times daily under your tongue the day before your treatment and continue taking them four times daily for two to three days after your treatment. If you get a small bruise, continue taking Arnica until the bruising is gone. You can also apply Calendula ointment to the bruise twice a day. The injection sites are first cleaned with alcohol. We apply a specially compounded topical anesthetic cream to these areas. This numbing cream numb works exceptionally well and also decreases the chance of bruising because it constricts blood vessels. When there is sufficient anesthetic effect, the injection sites are further cooled with ice and then cleaned again with alcohol. Following the injections, direct pressure is applied to avoid bruising at the injection sites.

4 STEPS TO BRUISE-FREE BOTOX®

1. Numb sufficiently with topical cream before injecting.

2. Apply ice packs before and after treatment.

3. Compress the injection site by applying pressure.

4. Take Arnica Montana sublingually before and after.

Forehead

Before treatment, the brow level, contour, and symmetry are noted. The position and shape of the eyelids are observed. The location and extent of horizontal forehead creases are noted. We ask you to raise your eyebrows and watch for dynamic furrows that may appear. We adjust the brow level and contour first with Botox®. Then we ask you to return in one week for a dose adjustment to treat any residual forehead creases that may be left. We will avoid treating your forehead if you have droopy or heavy upper eyelids and are using your frontalis forehead muscle to keep your eyes open and to maintain your peripheral vision.

We then observe the dynamic forehead folding by asking you to raise your brows. We can treat along the length of each horizontal furrow (at least one centimeter above the eyebrows to avoid any brow drooping). We can also treat segments to achieve a further balance of eyebrow level and contour shaping. If, after brow depressor muscle treatment, there is any segmental brow retraction—referred to as the "Dr. Spock" or "Jack Nicholson" effect—this can be corrected with one to two units injected into the wrinkle that is visible when you raise your eyebrows. Utilizing lower doses in the forehead yields a more natural result with an improved brow level and contour.

Glabella and Brow Depressors

We will observe you when you are not moving. If we see a deep furrow or two furrows, as in "your 11", we will suggest filling it with Restylane® or layered Perlane® and Restylane®. We then we will ask you to frown, feel your corrugator muscle, and inject the Botox® to the inside and outside of that muscle just above the bridge of the nose; this will also treat the medial brow depressors. Another injection is then given on the bridge of the nose, over the procerus muscle insertion. This is the muscle that causes a horizontal wrinkle on the bridge of the nose. These muscles are brow depressors. When they are relaxed and the elevating action of the frontalis forehead muscle is unopposed, the eyebrows can be successfully elevated.

Often a dose adjustment will have to be given in seven to ten days after the full effect of the Botox® is observed. We avoid giving too much and do not want you to have a frozen expression or a droopy brow.

Crow's Feet and Orbicularis Muscle

When we ask you to smile, the orbicularis muscle contracts and this will determine the extent and depth of any crow's feet. This will help us to determine exactly where to inject the Botox® and in how many places. Three to four injection sites per side, outside of the orbital bone, will soften crow's feet wrinkles safely and not exacerbate any lower lid laxity or cause any lower eyelid drooping. Injecting Botox® under the outside portion of the eyebrow will affect a portion of the orbicularis muscle and will segmentally relax it, allowing elevation of the tail of the brow. This is a critical step in brow shaping.

Lower Eyelids

Lower eyelid dynamic wrinkling and folding of the lower lid orbicularis muscle—which creates a roll under the lashes—can be treated with small doses of Botox®. To create a more opened eye, the lower eyelid orbicularis muscle can also be injected.

On occasion, lower lid wrinkling may persist or even be accentuated following crow's feet injections. This may be the result of muscle recruitment, when muscles not normally involved in smiling become overactive. Once a portion of the lower eyelid orbicularis muscle has been relaxed, the cheek smiling muscles can cause folds in the lower lid when you smile. This process may also be visible on the bridge of the nose, producing "bunny lines".

Nasolabial Folds

Using Botox® to treat your nasolabial groove is a distinct area of controversy. We prefer to fill the groove (Restylane®, Perlane®, Scultpra™) or, in patients with marked redundancy of the fold, to tighten the fold first (with Thermage® or laser resurfacing) and then fill in the residual fold (Restylane®, Perlane®, Radiesse™, Scultpra™). If you have a gummy smile—a smile that shows your gums above your upper teeth—then Botox® can be used to correct your smile and soften your nasolabial groove at the same time.

Vertical Upper Lip Lines

Upper lip vertical furrows, smokers' lines, and lipstick bleeding may be cautiously treated with one to two units of Botox® to each side of the upper lip, spaced one centimeter from the midline and one centimeter apart. While this is a wonderfully effective technique, too much Botox® or slight misplacement can give you an asymmetric smile. We also warn our patients that this technique can affect their whistling (like our patient who temporarily lost her dog because she could not whistle) or their ability to play a wind instrument. Because of the small doses used, successful outcomes rarely last longer than two months. However, this technique works well in combination with fillers (Restylane®, Restylane® Fine Lines, CosmoDerm®) and as a pretreatment for laser resurfacing.

Marionette lines (Melo-Mental folds, oral commissures)

This multi-contoured area is difficult to treat completely with any single modality. A combination of Botox® to the muscle that pulls the corners of the mouth down and thicker fillers like Perlane® or Sculptra®, will subtly elevate the corners of the mouth and allow more efficient filling of the residual depression. When we ask you to show us your lower teeth, we will be able to feel the muscle. By extending a straight line from the nasolabial fold to the border of the jay, we can identify the just where we have to place the Botox®. If the injection is given too close to the chin, the mentalis muscle can be affected and you may have difficulty lowering your lower lip. If the injection is given too close to the lower lip, the orbicularis oris may be affected, and the lower lip may not function properly, causing you to drool.

If your Botox® treatments give you a result that you are not happy with, the good news is that the effect is temporary and your muscles will return to normal in about a month or two.

COMBINATION THERAPIES

The beauty of combination therapies is that the end result is always greater than the effects of each individual treatment.

There are several areas in the face where Botox® can give improved and longer lasting results when combined with fillers and other treatment modalities.

Botulinum toxin with fillers to treat the glabellar crease

If you have deep static furrows—"your 11"—that persist even at rest, filling them gives immediate improvement that is accentuated after the Botox® takes effect. The improvement lasts longer (six to twelve months) than when either Botox® or fillers are used alone.

Botulinum toxin with fillers to treat the marionette lines (melo-mental grooves, oral commissures)

Filling agents make these grooves less noticeable. Botox® to the depressor anguli oris muscles will elevate the corners of the mouth and diminish the muscle ridge descending from the corner of the mouth. This will allow more complete filling and a more satisfying result with a thicker filling agent (Perlane®, Sculptra®)

Pretreatment for IPL (Intense Pulsed Light)

IPL is an effective treatment for broken capillaries, redness, rosacea, brown spots, and skin texture. All of our treatments that improve the quality and texture of the skin will make the Botox® and the filler effects more striking. However, a secondary Botox® effect results in improvement greater than that achieved by either Botox® or IPL on their own. Similarly, Botox® appears to enhance the skin texture improvement achieved with non-ablative lasers as well. In all likelihood, Botox® will also augment the effects of non-thermal, non-ablative photomodulation utilizing light-emitting diodes (LED's).

Pretreatment for laser resurfacing

Using botulinum toxin one to two weeks before laser resurfacing has become standard procedure. Its effect is crucial during the period of collagen remodeling. Under ideal circumstances, we treat patients two weeks before the laser resurfacing procedure. This gives use an opportunity for additional adjustments if necessary before laser resurfacing.

The principle is similar to trying to remove pleats from a pair of trousers. You have to release the pleat before you press the pants, otherwise the pleat will remain.

Laser resurfacing of the eyelids or face will tighten and lift the skin, removing wrinkles and creating new collagen. If the eyelid and facial muscles have been relaxed with Botox® while the new collagen is being formed, the result will be a much smoother skin. On the other hand, if the eyelid and facial muscles have not been relaxed with Botox® before the formation of new collagen begins, and these muscles are in constant movement, the new collagen will not be as smooth.

The use of botulinum toxin has evolved from a localized

stand alone therapeutic miracle that magically diminished dynamic lines, furrows, and wrinkles from the face and eyelids, to an integral preparatory step for our facial and eyelid rejuvenation techniques. As we explore the delicate relationships and the balance of the facial musculature, more indications and potential uses of Botox® will emerge.

Erika's Facial Rejuvenation

When we first met Erika, she was an attractive women with magnificent bone structure but skin that showed signs of too much sun and smoking. We discussed the folds that she did not like and the less than perfect quality of her skin. We outlined a course of action, including stopping smoking and all the non-invasive modalities— Botox®, Restylane®, IPL, Thermage®—as well as laser resurfacing and laser blepharoplasty. But Erika really was not motivated enough to proceed. Two years later she came back to see us. Her facial skin had not changed much, but now she was motivated. She had just been diagnosed with lung cancer and wanted to look as good as possible before she began her cancer therapy. On the same day we relaxed her frown lines, smile creases, and her marionette lines with Botox®, we filled in her sunken cheeks with Sculptra®. We softened the lines around her lips and mouth with Restylane®, Perlane®, and CosmoPlast®. She left the office looking great and feeling much better, psychologically prepare for the journey ahead of her.

INNOVATIVE USES FOR BOTULINUM TOXIN

Each new location and each new application for Botox® is a logical development emanating from the understanding of how Botox® works and how the facial muscles work in their delicate balance. What is initially an innovation, soon becomes standard practice. A few short years ago raising the corners of the mouth was a new innovation and now it is one of our most popular treatments.

What Is Coming Next?

Just as we have prepared our laser resurfacing patients with Botox®, we now prepare our Thermage® patients with Botox® as well. The **BZ Lift** (patent pending) treats the muscles that pull down the brows, causing brow ptosis and drooping brows, and also treats the muscles that pull down the lower face, causing sagging of the jowls, allowing Thermage® treatments to be more effective. The **BZ Lift** is completed with fillers to support and fill the facial struc- tures. We are investigating the advantages of using Botox® with Reloxan®.

CHAPTER 10

New & Improved Methods of Light Source & Radio Frequency Skin Tightening

Choices in lasers today range from the deep ablative models to new innovations that produce new collagen and tighten loose skin.

Skin rejuvenation includes removing vascular and pigmented lesions, improving skin texture and resilience, and reducing fine facial wrinkles. We will review the resurfacing and skin tightening options that are available, explain how these devices work, which ones we like, and why we like them.

Intense pulse light gives good results for vascular, pigmented lesions and skin texture. Photo Dynamic Therapy (equivalent to three to four IPL sessions) diminishes precancerous areas (actinic keratoses) and even superficial skin cancers. Thermage® radiofrequency technology is primarily a technique for lifting and tightening, not for wrinkle or pigment reduction. The same holds true for Orion's ST handpiece and Lumenis' Aluma which also tighten the deeper layers of the skin. Non-ablative lasers like the Cool Touch™ II improve texture and fine wrinkling, but do not improve pigment.

Carbon dioxide laser resurfacing literally changed the face of facial skin rejuvenation and is the gold standard. Carbon dioxide laser resurfacing lifts, smoothes, tightens, and improves pigment. The standard techniques that have been used until now require a prolonged recovery time. The first two weeks require constant care, but the results can be great. Occasionally there is a period of increased pigmentation following laser resurfacing (transient post-inflammatory hyperpigmentation) and rarely, in selected individuals, there can be loss of skin pigmentation (hypopigmentation). Now CO2 Lite™ (Lumenis) is catching on. The carbon dioxide laser is used on its lowest power settings. Multiple treatment sessions are necessary, but the downtime is minimal. Fraxel™ (Reliant) offers another option. It resurfaces tiny spots and allows the untreated areas in between the spots to stimulate rapid healing. The downtime with Fraxel™ is also minimal, but at least four sessions are needed, and the results are less dramatic than carbon dioxide laser resurfacing.

Our preferred technique now is to perform a Thermage® treatment for lifting and tightening followed by a TCA peel, PDT, or CO2 Lite™ for texture and pigment correction. We reserve full face ablative CO2 laser resurfacing for patients with severe photodamage.

ABLATIVE LASERS—WHERE IT ALL BEGAN

Carbon Dioxide

In the early 1990's carbon dioxide laser resurfacing provided a breakthrough in facial rejuvenation—never before had such dramatic results been achieved. Facial tightening, lifting, and smoothing that surpassed any cold steel surgical technique was finally possible. Skin resurfacing techniques have come a long way since the first days of carbon dioxide lasers. However, in most cases, one to two weeks for initial healing and three to six months for the pinkness to fade are necessary following full face CO2 laser resurfacing. There are some preliminary indications that the use of LED's (light emitting diodes) before and after the procedure may help. And there are now alternative options that can be offered minimizing the downtime.

The tissue target for the carbon dioxide laser is water. Skin cells are composed primarily of water. The water within the most superficial cells of the skin absorbs the laser energy and the cells are heated up until they are vaporized or ablated. So it is only the most superficial cells of the epidermis that are vaporized with laser resurfacing. If there is extreme sun damage and deep wrinkling, then more than one pass of the laser is required to smooth the wrinkles and tighten the skin. Each pass of the laser heats up the deeper layers of the skin a little more and causes more tightening. The more times the laser is passed over the tissue, the more tissue tightening there is, but the longer time that is necessary for healing. The power of each laser application can also be varied, using lower power on the thin eyelid skin, and higher power on the face. Extra passes can be applied to the areas of most photodamage like the upper lip and nose. CO_2 laser resurfacing can cause 30 to 50 percent skin shrinkage and dramatically reduce deeper wrinkles.

Laser Blepharoplasty

We also use the carbon dioxide laser instead of a scalpel to perform blepharoplasty. Because it seals blood vessels, the procedure can be performed with minimal bruising and faster healing.

While this technique can provide dramatic improvement beyond what most other procedures can provide, the post-operative course is often more than many patients are willing to accept.

POTENTIAL DRAWBACKS OF LASER RESURFACING

• Pink skin may last for several months.

• Increased skin pigmentation (usually transient)

• Decreased skin pigmentation with possible demarcation lines between the untreated and treated areas.

• Changes in skin texture.

• Milia (tiny white bumps like what are sometimes seen on a baby's bottom)

- Prophylactic bacterial antibiotics and anti-herpetic medication to prevent infections and cold sores

- Medication for calming pigment (hydroquinone)

- Medication for stimulating more rapid healing (retinoids)

- Discontinue Accutane® for at least one year before treatment

- If there is looseness of the lower eyelid margin or tendon, it may need to be tightened to avoid retraction or drooping of the lower eyelid

Carbon Dioxide Laser Care

During the first week following full face CO2 laser resurfacing, there are many hours of cleansing and creaming. Our standard protocol consists of twice daily vinegar washes (One tablespoon of white vinegar in four cups of lukewarm water) followed by applications of CU3 copper peptide cream four times daily. During the second post-operative week, Aquaphor ointment is applied every two hours during the day. After the second week you can again venture outside, using camouflage make-up that will protect your resurfaced skin from the sun. You can continue using Aquaphor whenever your skin feels dry. After four weeks you can begin using a lighter moisturizer (B+Z crystal C gel) and a transparent zinc oxide sun block and makeup containing sun block.

After ablative resurfacing, your skin will be exceptionally sensitive. DO NOT USE any skincare products, herbs, or botanicals unless we approve them first. You will begin taking anti-viral medication, one day pre-operatively and continue taking it for one to two weeks post-operatively until the surface of your skin is completely healed.

Upper and Lower Laser Eyelift and Carbon Dioxide Laser Skin Resurfacing

When we met 45-year old Olga, she complained of looking tired all the time. She had heavy upper eyelid folds that rested on her lashes and her lower lids had a slight fat bulge that created the appearance of dark circles. Her facial skin was blotchy with irregular pigmentation, broken capillaries and poor elasticity, creating a wrinkled appearance.

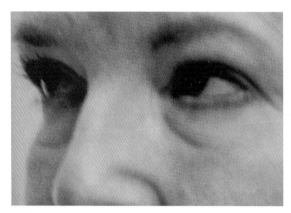

Before

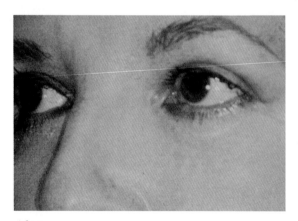

After

A carbon dioxide laser was used to remove a small amount of upper eyelid skin and shrink the fat pockets of the upper lid. To tighten and smooth the eyelid skin, a computer pattern generator was used to guide the laser as it resurfaced the skin and helped Olga's body manufacture new collagen. Some of the fat from the lower lid was melted to reduce the puffiness; this fat was then shifted into the indented areas to create a youthful look. The final result was a natural one, with no incisions to the skin. Both Olga and her husband were thrilled.

Upper and Lower Laser Eyelift
with Muscle Adjustments

36-year old Sherri looked older than her age because her upper eyelid muscles were out of place. Frequent allergy attacks caused her eyelids to swell. Recurrent swelling made her upper eyelid muscles detach, or "disinsert", causing the eyelids to droop. A second problem was lower eyelids that hung too low and didn't cover enough of her eye, thus exposing too much white (sclera). If we merely raised her upper lids without raising the lower lids, her eyes would be in a perpetual stare.

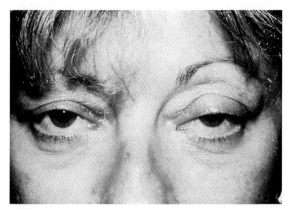

Before

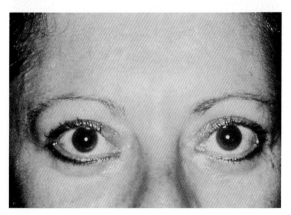

After

We reattached her upper eyelid muscles to the correct position, melted some extra eyelid fat, and trimmed the skin to restore a natural fold. Extra lower eyelid fat was melted (from the inside of the eyelid), without cutting the skin, and the surrounding support muscles were tightened to raise the border of the lower lid.

Upper and Lower Laser Eyelift
and Laser Skin Resurfacing

Helmut just turned 60. He spent many years pursuing an athletic life in the sun. He was looking for a new wife and although he was fit and energetic, he felt he looked too old. His upper lids were heavy, lower lids saggy, and he was unhappy with the quality and texture of his skin.

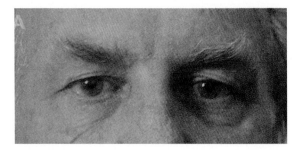

Before

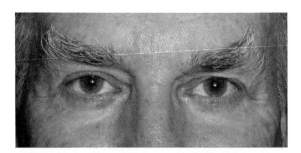

After

Removal of some eyelid skin, and an upper eyelid incision internal brow suspension, added support to his brows and lifted his upper lids. Support was added to the lower lid tendons and the entire face, including the lower lids, was resurfaced with the carbon dioxide laser. Men are excellent candidates for cosmetic eyelid procedures, although the techniques used for men are different than women.

Upper Eyelid Creases

Toshi, a 32-year old Japanese woman, wanted both sides of her face to look the same. Her right upper lid had two different creases and folds; her left upper lid had one low crease and one fold. Everyone wants both sides of their faces to look the same. Unfortunately, perfect symmetry rarely occurs in nature.

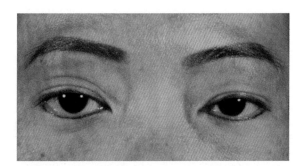

Before

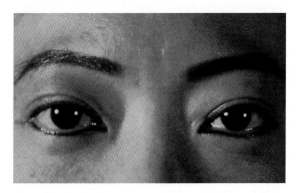

After

The symmetry, position, depth, and contour of the upper eyelid crease was corrected by reattaching the eyelid muscles to the skin at the same level on each side. This is a particular problem for the Asian patient. Toshi was very pleased with the result.

Upper and Lower Laser Eyelift with Adjustment of Lower Lid Support Tendon Restores Lower Lid Contour

African and African-American skin heals differently than Caucasian. Keloids and exuberant scarring can occur on the body, but rarely on eyelid skin. Eyelift procedures can be performed on this group with excellent results and minimal risk. 57 year old Charmee was troubled by heavy upper eyelids and the appearance of her lower lids. She wanted to appear more youthful.

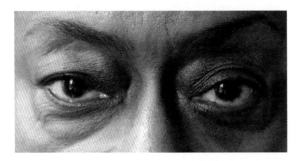

Before

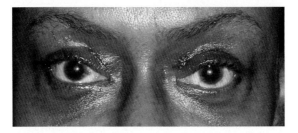

After

We were able to create a youthful appearance by removing a small amount of upper eyelid skin, melting and reshaping her upper eyelid fatty tissue, and reshaping and shifting the fatty tissue of her lower eyelid. Finally, the tendons that support her lower eyelids were lifted. Laser eyelifts are effective for patients of all skin types.

Treatment of Lower Eyelid Pigmentation with Beautif-Eye Nourishing Cream, Alpha Hydroxy Acid Peels, and CO2Cellulair™

African-American skin can be very sensitive. Any kind of irritation or inflammation can sometimes make it darker. 42 year old Doris always remembered dark under eye circles. However, her circles became worse after an allergy attack.

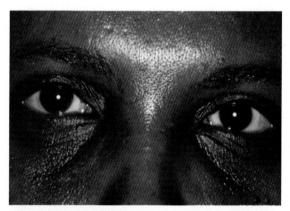

Before

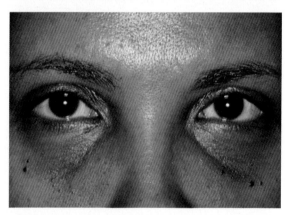

After

The quality, texture, and pigmentation of the facial skin, was restored with a combination of treatments, including CO2 Cellulaire, gentle AHA peels, and B+Z Beautif-Eye Cream. The treatment took five weeks; results were visible after the second week. Excellent improvement was noted on the lower eyelid pigmentation.

Eyeliner Micropigmentation

59 year old Rebecca dreamed of waking in the morning, ready to go, and having the appearance of thick eyelashes.

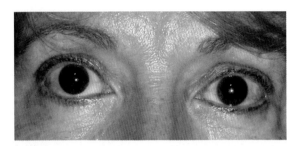

Before

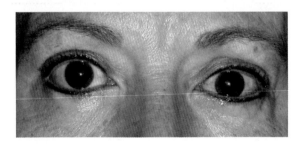

After

Micropigmentation (semi-permanent makeup) brought Rebecca's eyes to life and added definition. Using a surgical magnifying glass, tiny dots of pigment are placed between the lashes to create a thick appearance. The procedure takes forty-five minutes and needs to be touched up after one month. The results last for three years. This method is effective to enhance pale or sparse eyelashes and eyebrows and to fill in areas where hair is missing. For special occasions, makeup can be applied over the micropigmentation.

Treatment of "Number 11" Brow Furrows with Restylane® and Botulinum Toxin

Always serious and frequently frowning, 32-year old Anna had deep furrows between the brows that were apparent even when she was not frowning. Botox® improved the situation but did not result in a complete correction.

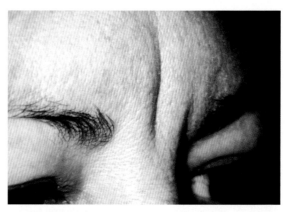

Before

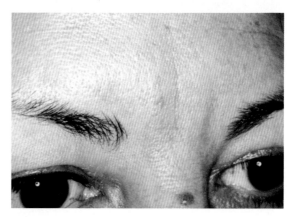

After

Botox® was used to relax the muscles in the area between the brows and Restylane® was used to fill in the grooves. Combining the two treatments gives a complete and long lasting result. The correction lasted for one year. Anna has maintained the result with Botox® injections three times a year and Restylane® once a year.

The BZ Lift Using Thermage® and Botox®

Barbara wanted to celebrate her 60th birthday by rejuvenating her face in a subtle, natural way. She wanted a lift to her cheekbones and a more defined jawline. The procedures selected for her would take a few weeks so she happily scheduled with us on the way to a weekly karate class.

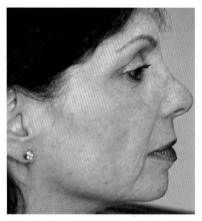

Before

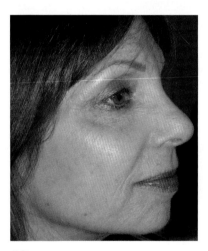

After

First we used Botox® to elevate the corners of the mouth and relax the muscles that pulled down her jawline. The following week, Thermage® was used to tighten the skin over the cheekbones and jawline and to decrease the folds alongside the nose. Two weeks later Sculptra® was used to plump up the indented areas around her mouth. The result lifted her midface area, with better cheek contour and a clean jawline. This non-surgical combination treatment is known as the "BZ Lift".

Dramatic Results with Full Face Laser Resurfacing

48-year old Caroline looked years older than her chronological age with delicate skin that showed all her wrinkles, sun damage, a saggy jawline, and lipstick "bleed" lines above her upper lip.

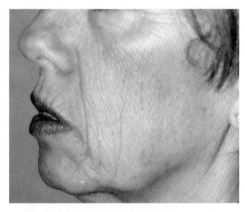

Before

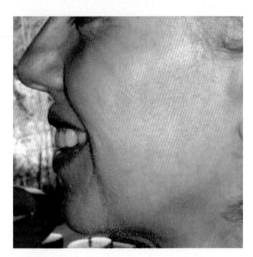

After

It is hard to believe that this is the same patient before and after a full face treatment with carbon dioxide laser resurfacing. The skin is tighter and the smoothing and lifting effects are remarkable. Wrinkles are gone - precancerous skin lesions disappear—Botox® was used to treat the muscles that pull down the side of the mouth and lower face. No other procedure can duplicate the extent of this improvement. However, it takes patience. Most patients are not comfortable with public appearances for two weeks; coverup makeup is generally used for blotchiness for several months and no sun is allowed. The results are worth the effort and new skin collagen that forms after this procedure will last for decades.

Treatment of the Peri-Oral Area
with Botox®, Thermage®, and Sculptra®

59-year old Joan did not like the effects of aging around her mouth, which included downward shadows, marionette lines, and extra folds.

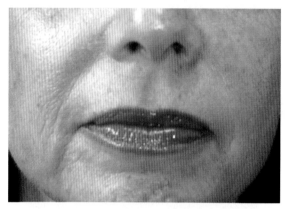

Before

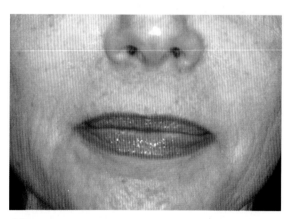

After

Combination therapies produced a softer, more pleasing appearance. Botox® was used to relax the muscles that pull down the sides of the mouth. Two weeks later Thermage® was used to tighten the cheek folds. And a month later, Sculptra® was used to decrease the marionette lines.

Treatment with B+Z Clarifying Lotion, AHA Peels, and Intense Pulsed Light (IPL)

Liz was 37 years old and still had acne breakouts. Red spots remained for approximately a week and then turned brown. Sometimes they left scars so deep that when Liz tanned, the spots showed white.

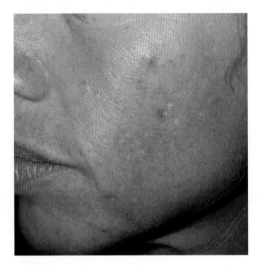

Before

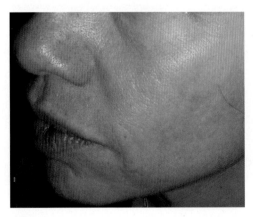

After

The combination of advanced skin care products and in-office treatments improved the skin texture and pigmentation dramatically. To control acne, reduce the brown and red spots, and improve skin texture, we prescribed nightly treatments of B+Z clarifying lotion, weekly AHA peels, and a monthly IPL treatment.

Treating Sun Damaged Skin with Photodynamic Therapy (PDT) with Levulan, Sculptra®, and Radiesse®

Claire had suffered with acne scars since she was a teenager. To improve her appearance, she became a sun worshipper. By the age of 32, her acne scars had not improved and she had developed sun damaged skin.

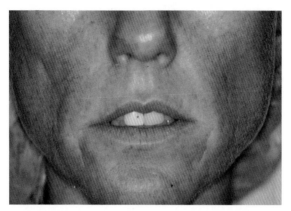

Before

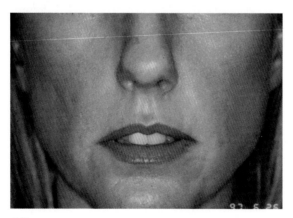

After

We achieved an impressive improvement of sun damaged skin by using photodynamic therapy. Areas of skin irregularity and depressions were effectively filled with Sculptra® and Radiesse®. Her newly improved skin reflected the translucent quality of her preteen years.

Correcting Nasal Deformities with Restylane®
Rhinoplasty and Perlane Augmentation

41-year old Vickie had endured 5 nasal surgeries. Surgeons were hesitant to perform another surgical procedure.

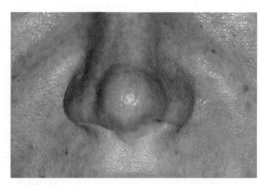

Before

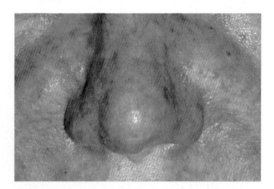

After

Restylane®, and other filling agents, can correct nasal deformities without surgery, as well as filling in wrinkles and facial folds. The first reported Restylane® rhinoplasty was performed on Vickie, rebuilding and recontouring her nose gradually over several months and finally augmenting the effect with layers of Perlane.

Upper Lip Augmentation with Restylane®

32-year old Vanessa felt that her upper lip was too thin and lacked definition. She wanted her lips to be fuller and in balance with the rest of her facial features.

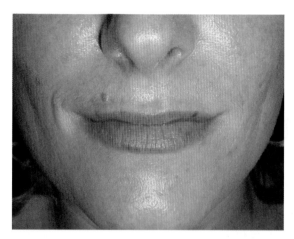

Before

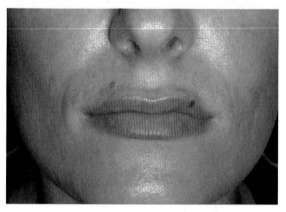

After

Like all of the procedures that we perform, each patient is evaluated on an individual basis. The shape, contour, and volume of the upper and lower lips need to be adjusted to create a desired effect. Restylane® was used to enhance the upper lip border and overall contour of the lip.

Lip and Perioral Rejuvenation with Botox®, Restylane®, Thermage® and Micropigmentation

56-year old Andrea felt that her lips had diminished in size and that with age, her face seemed longer. Just as eyes dominate the upper face, the mouth dominates the lower face and is a major factor in overall appearance.

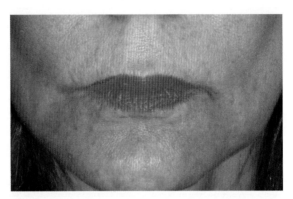

Before

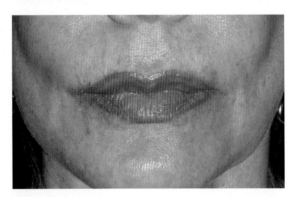

After

Combining different treatments can create a dramatic improvement. We have relaxed the muscles that pull down the corners of the mouth with Botox®, tightened the lower face with Thermage®, enhanced the volume of the lip with Restylane®, and created a beautifully pigmented lip line with micropigmentation. Some patients only need to enhance their lips by increasing volume, while others need to add missing pigment or expand the area of the pigmentation. When the pigmented area is increased, the lips need fairly little plumping.

ERBIUM:YAG

The erbium:yttrium-aluminum-garnet (Er:YAG) laser emits laser energy in the mid-infrared light spectrum. This wavelength has ten to fifteen times more affinity for water than the carbon dioxide (CO_2) laser. Because its wavelength is at the peak of water absorption, it is a true epidermal ablation laser, which means that it works more superficially.

The erbium laser flattens the wrinkles but does not create much heat. It is the heat that creates the tightening effect of the CO_2 laser, but also the long-lasting pinkness. Generally, the Erbium:YAG laser needs a shorter recovery time and results in less pinkness. This technology gained wide acceptance as the second cousin to Carbon Dioxide, without the prolonged time necessary for healing. It works well on fine lines and wrinkles, mild sun damage, and scars. Since skin cells are predominantly water, the laser energy is absorbed by the first cells it touches. There is little heat damage to the deeper layers of the skin.

Because the Er:YAG laser applications are more superficial (three passes of the erbium are roughly equivalent to one pass of the CO_2 laser), there is more rapid healing. This laser is also well suited for resurfacing the delicate eyelid skin.

Erbium:YAG Laser Care

Cleansing and lubrication are key. Although the recovery time from Er:YAG treatments are significantly less than following CO_2 laser resurfacing, the same general principles apply. Showering and shampooing with baby shampoo twice daily and using a vinegar face wash twice daily during the first week will keep the face clean and minimize crusting. After the first week, the face should be cleansed twice daily with B + Z white cleanser and moisturized with B + Z Lipocel Cream Moist. Once healing is complete, morning and evening eyelid cleansing with B+Z non-alcoholic toner and light moisturizing with B + Z crystal C gel is recommended for maintenance care.

Intense sun protection is essential for all patients during the first eight to twelve weeks following the procedure. Zinc oxide is a total physical sun block and a soothing topical agent. We encourage our patients to use it for at least two weeks before they begin using makeup with an SPF15. For treatments of the entire face, a course of antibiotics is begun one day pre-operatively and continued until the skin is completely healed in about one week. We have also begun studies using red and infrared LED's (light emitting diodes) to accelerate healing and diminish redness more quickly.

The Er:YAG laser may be used very cautiously, with lower powers, on darker skin types (Fitzpatrick III and IV). More darkly pigmented patients will frequently heal with a short period of skin darkening (post-inflammatory hyperpigmentation) beginning two to four weeks after the procedure. Topical cortisone creams will help this pass more quickly.

NON-ABLATIVE LASERS AND LIGHT SOURCES

Non-ablative treatment of deep wrinkles remains a difficult challenge in aesthetic medicine; however each generation of devices offers better results.

The key advantages of non-ablative (not requiring external healing) therapies are that they do not produce the downtime of deeper treatments. Non-ablative broadband light and laser devices have become more popular in recent years. The intense pulsed light (IPL) was introduced in the mid-1990's and is a well-recognized treatment option for photoaging, redness, veins, rough texture, and mottled pigmentation.

Non-ablative laser devices emit energy in a single (coherent) wavelength within the infrared spectrum aimed at a target tissue within each skin cell. The heat generated by this interaction causes a mild heat (thermal) injury within the skin, and as a result, new collagen formation is promoted as part of the repair process. This creates a subtle improvement in fine wrinkling and skin texture.

We commonly use vascular lasers to treat dilated blood vessels. The blood pigment selectively absorbs the energy. Light energy is converted to heat, which damages the vessel walls.

THE INCREDIBLE IPL

By contrast, IPL is a non-coherent (more than one wave length of light) device, which emits a spectrum of larger wavelengths. We are able to control the range of light wavelengths and the power that is emitted so we can safely treat without downtime. This process of using a series of no downtime light therapy sessions is called photorejuvenation.

We can even treat some patients of darker skin types (Fitzpatrick III). With IPL, we can target blood vessels as well as sun spots. Usually three to five treatments are necessary to get the maximum effect. New collagen formation and improvement of skin texture are secondary effects. Cooling systems and cool gels used with these devices allow for their safe use, protecting the superficial layers of your skin while you are being treated. IPL treatments show dramatic results, are low-risk, and have minimal downtime, which is what our patients want.

We have been using the IPL™ Quantum SR (Lumenis) and the Orion device with great results. Both devices use a flash-lamp—a type of giant flash so bright that you will have to wear goggles when you are being treated. The bright flash is shocking, but not really uncomfortable, causing only a slight burning sensation.

How can broken capillaries be treated?

One of the most frequently requested procedures is elimination of broken capillaries of the face, chest, and legs. In order to treat blood vessels by light energy, the blood vessel pigment absorbs a specific wave length of light and is destroyed. IPL is very useful for this purpose.

Broken capillaries on the face are generally more responsive to IPL treatment than those on the legs because of thinner overlying skin and thinner vessel walls on the face, which make them more susceptible to thermal damage.

After only three IPL treatments, broken capillaries on the face have a 95 percent resolution rate.

The use of ice-cold cooling gel makes the IPL procedure more comfortable. Within seconds after a treatment, blood vessels darken and turn reddish-blue. This coloration can travel slightly beyond the treated area, as the heat energy is conducted along the vessel. There can be mild redness following treatment and multiple sessions are required for best results.

Treating Age Spots

Solar lentigines, known as "sun spots," "age spots," and "liver spots" are another characteristic of photoaging. These gradually appear as light and dark brown round smooth colored patches on the cheeks and forehead. Often mistaken for moles, they can be effectively treated with IPL devices. Within twenty-four to forty-eight hours after treatment, the spots take on a darker and crusty appearance that will spontaneously peel away over a five to six day period. This can be facilitated by using microdermabrasion on the second day after IPL treatment.

PHOTODYNAMIC THERAPY

Photodynamic therapy (PDT)—lotion plus light—marries a strong light with a chemical that absorbs light energy. Originally created as a treatment for precancerous actinic keratoses and superficial skin cancers (basal cell carcinomas) as well, it now impresses all of us as an effective treatment for the splotchy pigmentation of photoaging, large pores, prominent oil glands, and acne. PDT works when the light interacts with the Levulan™ (Kerastick®, DUSA) that has been applied to the skin. The interaction creates a reactive form of oxygen that creates a cellular reaction. The longer this colorless dye is left on the skin, the more intense the response and the longer the time needed for healing. One hour seems just long enough to create an impressive effect without too much downtime. One PDT session is the equivalent of three to four IPL sessions. This technology is rapidly adding another dimension to our non-invasive menu.

The actual process begins by thoroughly cleansing the skin using acetone or alcohol to enable the colorless aminolevulinic acid to penetrate the skin. After the Levulan™ has been left on the skin for one hour, it is washed off, and then your face is exposed to a light source—either IPL or a blue light (Blu U). There can be a mild stinging or burning sensation during the treatment. When the treatment is complete is it critical for you stay out of the sun on your way home from the office to avoid an extreme sunburn. Normally you will be red and peeling for four to five days.

Improving Skin Texture and Pigmentation

Intense pulsed light (IPL) has been our workhorse for diminishing pigmentation, broken capillaries, and redness. Although improvement in skin texture is not its primary function, these changes do occur. We currently use two different IPL machines—Quantum by Lumenis for pigment (560 filter) and broken capillaries (590 filter). We use the 570 Orion filter for brown and red. IPL treatments also help acne because it shuts down sebaceous glands in the skin. This action also decreases pore size, but the effect only lasts about three months and will have to be repeated.

Light Emitting Diodes

Light emitting diodes (LEDs)—Gentle Waves® and Omni-Lux—enhance the results of IPL. LED photomodulation uses low energy, nonlaser, nonthermal, light energy to stimulate mitochondrial activity, increase collagen and fibroblast production, and decrease collagenase. What this means is that this form of light treatment stimulates new collagen and decreases the enzyme that breaks down collagen. The treatment lasts fifty seconds and is given once a week for eight weeks. There are several other LED therapies (Omnilux) that use red and yellow light. Early studies indicate that these treatments (twenty minutes each week, using yellow on one week and red on the next) can accelerate healing after deeper laser therapies.

Nd:YAG (Non-ablative neodynium:yttrium-aluminum-garnet) lasers create secondary collagen regrowth while protecting the skin surface with a cryogen spray. Our experience with the Cool Touch™ II (Cutera, Brisbane, California) has been generally good for mild wrinkling and acne scarring. They have seen substantial improvement after four to six monthly treatments. The depth of the treatment can be varied, applying the cooling spray immediately following each laser pulse (post-cooling). We use one precooling and two post-cooling applications in our treatment sessions. Redness is typically gone within thirty minutes.

The more sun damage you have, the more aggressive treatment is necessary. This is the art of laser resurfacing; knowing what to use when and where.

Although recovery time is minimal, the drawbacks of using Cool Touch lasers are the discomfort during the procedure, the subtlety of the improvement, and the number of sessions required. As with all non-ablative laser therapies for skin texture, they must be combined with additional therapies to improve pigment and capillaries.

Non-ablative laser therapies are theoretically very useful, but they require many treatments and the effects are not so dramatic. We prefer to use our most effective triad of therapies—Botox®, Thermage®, and IPL (with or without PDT).

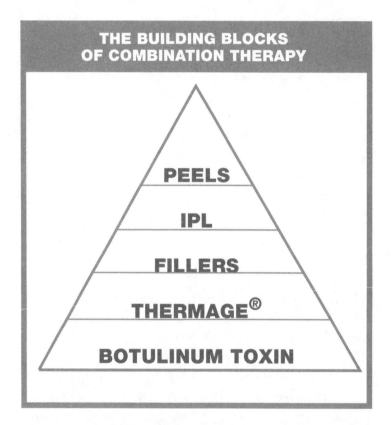

THE BUILDING BLOCKS OF COMBINATION THERAPY

PEELS

IPL

FILLERS

THERMAGE®

BOTULINUM TOXIN

RADIOFREQUENCY—THE NEXT GENERATION

Expectations are so high that there is no room for complications when you are performing minimally invasive cosmetic techniques.

THERMAGE: THE OVERVIEW

- Radio frequency energy heats deeper layers of skin and subcutaneous support tissue while the surface of the skin is cooled.

- Effect begins at the end of the treatment, and improves over the next 3-6 months.

- One treatment often works, but multiple sessions sometimes advised after 3 months.

- Multiple lower-power passes each session, varying the number of pulses:

  Mid- and lower face: 300-500 pulses
  Neck: 100-200 pulses
  Browlift (pretreated with Botulinum toxin): 100-200 pulses
  Arms: 300-600 pulses
  Abdomen: 600-900 pulses
  Buttocks: 600-900 pulses

- Discomfort moderate

- Temporary flushing, gone in 10-15 minutes; mild soreness.

Although the use of radiofrequency energy is a relatively new concept in aesthetic medicine, we have been using it for twenty-five years. The first radiofrequency technology we worked with utilized very fine wires mounted on a stylus, like a pen. We used it to make fine incisions and to melt fat. This represented a great advance. Before the advent of the carbon dioxide laser, we used it for all of our surgical procedures. The CO_2 laser expanded the techniques of bloodless surgery, and made them even more effective. We still use this radiofrequency instrumentation for scarless removal of moles and other growths of the face and body, and it is our preferred method. A looped electrode can shave off a mole one layer at a time, so that no stitches are necessary and the area becomes completely flat, without leaving a scar.

A new generation of instrumentation utilizing radiofrequency energy has introduced the possibility of skin tightening without downtime. By tightening the skin's surface, we have seen improvement of the skin folds and acne scarring. This technology delivers RF energy for non-ablative tissue tightening while cooling the skin. Heating the skin can shrink collagen, and stimulate tissue remodeling. The result is collagen contraction and tissue tightening followed by new collagen production over time. During the past three years, we have been using radiofrequency energy to lift and tighten the face and neck (and even skin on the arms and thighs). This can be accomplished without causing redness or visible after effects on the skin surface. And although its primary use is not for reducing facial wrinkles, it does improve skin texture.

RF energy heats the deeper layers of the skin and the supporting tissues. In the past this procedure has been very uncomfortable due to a high depth of penetration and heating. This has much improved as we have worked with the technology. The discomfort has been decreased with more rapid treatment tips, lower power settings, and a new treatment protocol. Now, less than half of our patients take any oral pain medication before their treatment.

We begin the procedure by determining the energy level that each patient can tolerate. After two passes over the area being treated at this power, we lower the power setting. By passing over the tissue many times at lower energies, we are able to achieve a much more dramatic result with less discomfort.

Radio frequency skin tightening has evolved into an integral part of our facial rejuvenation protocol.

The response is gradual; it takes three to four months to see results after treatment. Patients may notice further improvement after a subsequent treatment six months later. The effects may include softer nasolabial folds, less visible jowls, sharper and tighter jaw line, and fewer neck wrinkles. Thermage® can also be used to target fat, especially under the chin, by precooling the tissue.

The early reports of depressed areas on the face following Thermage® treatments were due to high energy settings and occurred with the older, slower tips. With our new protocols of lower energy settings and multiple passes, these complications are a thing of the past. The procedure is far more tolerable, results are more predictable, there are fewer complications, and we are getting much more dramatic results.

The recent introduction of other non-invasive skin tightening modalities—like the Alma ST handpiece and Titan instrumentation that use infrared energy and work on the more superficial layers of the skin—may complement the deep tissue effects of Thermage. The new Aluma bipolar radio frequency instrument works differently, using suction on small areas of skin and then treating the skin from either side, and sounds promising and we await their clinical trials.

THE ALMA ST HANDPIECE: ADVANCED INFRARED TECHNOLOGY

- Uses infrared light source.
- Multiple passes (5-6) with each treatment session.
- No discomfort.
- At least 6 treatments 3-4 weeks apart.
- Do not see result at time of procedure.
- Augments Thermage® treatments.

Thermage® has become an important addition to our combination therapy menu of non-invasive facial rejuvenation.

A MOST EFFECTIVE COMBINATION THERAPY FOR NON-INVASIVE FACE-LIFTING– THE BZ LIFT (PATENT PENDING)	
STEP ONE	Botox® relaxation of muscles that pull down the face
STEP TWO	Thermage® for face lifting and tightening enhanced with CO2Cellulair™ and Alma ST
STEP THREE	Selected fillers for different facial areas
STEP FOUR	IPL/PDT for even pigmentation and reduction in pore size

Is that all there is?

There had been so much hype and discussion about how much the Thermage® procedure hurts that many patients are very surprised that the most current techniques are not very uncomfortable and that there is no discomfort afterwards.

Marjorie's Thermage® Experience

This brings to mind Marjorie, a lady in her late 50's who we had treated and was very pleased with the results of her Botox® treatments that had raised her brows, opened her eyelids, corrected the drooping of the corners of her mouth, and smoothed out the bands in her neck. She enjoyed the way that Restylane® and Perlane® had softened the lines that ran from her nose to her mouth and also supported the corners of her mouth. About one and one half years earlier we had performed the Thermage® procedure on her face (using an earlier technique with higher power settings and a slower tip), raising and tightening her cheeks, cleaning up and defining her jaw line. Her results were impressive, but she had found the procedure itself very uncomfortable. But now she returned to us to use Thermage® to tighten her neck skin. She had confidence that we would succeed in improving her neck appearance, but was somewhat apprehensive about how it would feel while we were performing the procedure. Using the new larger, faster tip and our new techniques using lower power settings, she did not find the procedure uncomfortable at all and was very surprised. When we were finished she said, "That's it? That's all there is?" She said that it reminded her of the conception of her first daughter. Of course we asked her to explain. "We were all virgins before we got married then, you know," she responded. "On our wedding night I was too nervous to do anything. But when we got to the Caribbean the next night, far away from home, I was a little more relaxed and let things happen. When we finished I asked 'Is that it? That's all there is?' Nine months later my first daughter was born."

Other RF Technologies

There are several other instruments that are also used for non-invasive lifting and tightening. The Titan and the Alma ST tip use infrared energy (instead of radio frequency energy) to heat the deeper layers of the skin. However this heating does not penetrate as deeply as the Thermage® deep tissue heating. Our experience with both types of instruments leads us to believe that perhaps more superficial heating during a second session may enhance the initial results of the Thermage® treatment.

COMBINATION THERAPIES

We pretreat patients with Botox® two weeks before their Thermage® procedure. If we are treating the forehead, we prepare the area with a chemical brow lift using Botox®. If we are treating the face and neck—**BZ Lift**—we prepare these areas by weakening the platysma with Botox®. In both cases relaxation of the muscles that depress the brow and the lower face in theory decrease resistance to collagen contraction and allow more efficient collagen remodeling. This can be supplemented with IPL and fillers to complete the **BZ Lift**.

The use of RF energy alone or in combination with other devices is likely to become an increasingly popular therapy in facial rejuvenation of the future.

COMBINATION THERAPY	RESULTS
BOTULINUM TOXIN & FILLERS	Combining the treatment of wrinkles due to expression (dynamic) as well as those due to loss of connective tissue (static). More complete and long lasting effect than either treatment by itself.
BOTULINUM TOXIN & IPL	Improve the surface of the skin while addressing the dynamic source of many facial wrinkles. Botox® also has an enhancing effect on IPL treatments.

IPLS & MICRODERMABRASION	Combining strategies to superficially resurface and tone the outer layers of skin with minimal downtime and risk. Using microdermabrasion the day after IPL speeds up the clearing of mottled pigmentation
MICRODERMABRASION & PEELS	Microdermabrasion & peels both address the outer layers of skin and polish it with different methods—harnessing chemical and mechanical techniques for improving outer skin appearance. Performing microdermabrasion first enhances the depth of the peel. Does not address wrinkles due to volume loss or facial expression.
SKINCARE, MICRODERMABRASION, PEELS, BOTOX®, FILLERS, IPL, CO2CELLULAIR™	Selecting the ideal skin treatment system for home use is essential for maximizing in-office treatments. B+Z homecare products "correct, protect, renew™"The better shape the skin is in, the greater the effect of other non-invasive therapies.
FILLERS & IPL, PDT	Fat or fillers are used to restore volume to the face, while IPL or PDT is used to tone and refine the texture of the outer layers of skin and improve its appearance.

OUR NEW INNOVATION—THE BZ LIFT

We have recently applied for a patent for a very effective combination therapy that we have introduced into our practices—the Bosniak+Zilkha lift or **BZ Lift**. It is a four step procedure that is completely non-invasive and without downtime. It is a combination of relaxing selected facial muscles, creating a new facial balance that will enhance facial tightening. Just as we use Botox® as a chemical brow-lift, we use Botox® in the **BZ Lift** to treat the neck muscle—the platysma—as a first step. This allows Step Two—deep skin and subcutaneous supportive layer tightening with Thermage®—to be more effective. To complete the effect, the skin is treated with IPL and residual surface irregularities are filled. The end result is an overall facial lifting and tightening, reduced sagging around the jaw line and less visible nasolabial folds, and improved skin quality and texture.

CHAPTER 11

Age Reversing Combination Therapies for Your Skin

Combining therapies can achieve a graceful natural result.

The overall appearance of aging skin is primarily related to the effects of sun exposure over time. Ultraviolet radiation damages structural components of the skin, chiefly collagen and elastic fibers. The appearance of the face is also affected by genetic factors, conditions such as rosacea, and the overall loss of elasticity associated with aging. Of course family traits ("My father has big lower eyelid bags" or "My mother has heavy eyelids.") and skin pigmentation will also affect how eyelids age. The skin around the eyes is extremely thin, making it more vulnerable to the sun's harsh effects. In fact, the lower eyelid can get quite a lot of sun exposure and is frequently the site of skin cancers. The upper lid is somewhat protected by the eyebrow and brow bone.

Signs of photoaging are becoming evident in younger individuals, especially those who regularly participate in outdoor recreational activities and have been exposed to increasingly high levels of UV radiation. Patients are now more accustomed to recognizing these signs and are more educated about the physiology of their skin.

Many Brazilians started off looking pale, and end up with skin the color of my mahogany desk from all the years in the sun. Even Botox® doesn't last as long in Brazil, because of cumulative sun exposure.

We provide a customized recommendation based on the individual needs and desires of our patients. There is no single formula for every patient, and fortunately, today there are many varied options. The recent development of safe, long-lasting, and readily available materials that add volume to facial structures and fill in static facial lines and furrows have given non-invasive facial rejuvenation an exciting new dimension. We have a wide array of non-surgical treatments that can dramatically improve your appearance, soften lines and wrinkles, plump facial contours, and control conditions such as acne, rosacea (flushing and broken capillaries), and melasma (spotchy pigmentation often called the mask of pregnancy).

When you are young, they are called freckles. As you get older, they are called age spots or keratoses. Actinic keratoses are flaky and hyperpigmented areas caused by sun exposure. They can become raised or even become precancerous. Hyperpigmentation simply means an excess of pigment in the skin. People who have darker skin types or who tan easily, have more pigment available to react to the sun and are more prone to form darker areas.

FITZPATRICK SKIN TYPES	
TYPE	DESCRIPTION
I	Never tans, always burns
II	Occasionally tans, usually burns
III	Often tans, sometimes burns
IV	Always tans, never burns
V	Rarely burns
VI	Never burns

Men and women with less pigment in their skin tend to form broken capillaries and small pigmented blotches and skin cancers. Dark and black skin also react negatively to sun exposure. Instead of developing skin cancers, they more commonly develop areas of darker pigmentation. This hyperpigmentation usually does not occur uniformly, but creates irregular patches of varying intensity.

If your complexion is marked by unsightly brown patches that never seem to go away, you are not alone. Pigmented skin can be difficult to treat, but we are working with new options. Our unique treatment programs combine customized topical formulations for daily home use, a full menu of individually mixed chemical peels, intense pulsed light (IPL), photodynamic therapy (PDT), non-ablative and resurfacing lasers, infra-red and Thermage® radiofrequency treatments when appropriate for the best results. The key to managing hyperpigmentation is the limitation of sun exposure. It is impossible to avoid the sun and UV exposure completely. While UVB is primarily responsible for sun burn, there are also UVA and UVC which can affect our skin. You are exposed to UVA and UVC even while driving in your car and when the sun is not shining. UVB rays have a shorter wavelength (290-320 nanometers) than UVA (320 to 400 nanometers). The longer UVA rays penetrate more deeply into the skin and break down collagen, elastic fibers, and cellular DNA, making the skin more vulnerable to free radical damage. UVA rays may be responsible for premature skin aging and for the development of skin cancers.

GLOGAU WRINKLE SCALE & TREATMENT MENU		
	SYMPTOMS	**TREATMENT**
LEVEL ONE	Minimal to no discoloration or wrinkling	Light Moisturizers (B+Z Crystal C gel) Sunscreen Topical and internal anti-oxidants
LEVEL TWO	Wrinkling with facial expression Lines around the mouth and eye areas Scattered pigment and broken capillaries	Sunscreen Moisturizers (Crystal C Gel, Satin Serum) B+Z sensitive clarifying lotion (with Kojic Acid and retinoids)

LEVEL TWO		Retinoids AHA peels Prophylactic Botox® to prevent progression of dynamic wrinkling
LEVEL THREE	Visible wrinkles at all times Noticeable discolorations	Sunscreen Moisturizers (Beautif-Eye™ Nourishing Cream, B+Z Crystal C Gel, B+Z Satin Serum) B+Z clarifying lotion (with hydroquinone and retinoids) AHA peels IPL series or PDT TCA peel Erbium laser peel
LEVEL FOUR	Widespread wrinkling Generalized skin discoloration Localized skin cancer	Sunscreen Moisturizers (Beautif-Eye™ Nourishing Cream, B+Z Crystal C Gel, B+Z Lipicel Cream Moist, B+Z Satin Serum) B+Z clarifying Lotion (extra strength retinoids + extra strength hydroquinone) PDT or TCA peel CO_2 laser resurfacing

Sunscreens must be applied as a thick paste and reapplied every two hours. Just because a sunscreen has an SPF 45 does not mean than it will give you enough protection if you put on a thin layer. Unless you slather it on thickly ten to fifteen minutes before you go outside, you may be getting only a small fraction of the advertised SPF. You also must make sure that your sunscreen has as physical block (some form of zinc oxide) to protect you from UVA and UVC as well as UVB. Our exposure to UVB occurs mostly during the peak hours of sunlight. On the other hand, UVA is present all day long irrespective of weather conditions—even when it is cloudy, foggy, or stormy. Most sunscreens only protect you from UVB. You also need anti-oxidant protection—both internal and topical. Take at least 1000mg of vitamin C daily after each meal (do not take this on an empty stomach) and 400 International Units of vitamin E daily. Blueberry and grapeseed extracts, Ginkgo Biloba, Glutathione, Quercetin and Selenium are also powerful anti-oxidants that should be taken daily. You should also apply topical vitamin C and vitamin E for more complete anti-oxidant protection.

Mexoryl®, a sunscreen available in Europe, appears to be more effective against UVA than any sunscreen we have in the US. Until it gets FDA approval, rely on physical sun block (containing zince oxide), internal and external anti-oxidants.

Treating Hyperpigmentation

Our first step to treat hyperpigmentation is to determine the cause. We perform a complete medical history and an evaluation of the skin as well as diagnostic tests, such as thyroid function tests hormone levels, and skin biopsies if necessary (for example, if there is an area of concern, a change in color, size, or thickness). Next, we eliminate the cause, if possible. For example, if a medication is causing skin darkening, discontinuing that medication may result in a clearing.

KEY CAUSES OF PIGMENT IRREGULARITES	
• Pregnancy	• Thyroid dysfunction
• Hormonal flux	• Certain medications
• Oral contraceptive use	• Nutritional deficiencies
• Genetic factors	

Melanocytes are the cells in the epidermis that produce melanin pigment. They respond to sunlight by producing more melanin to protect the keratinocytes (skin cells). Melanosomes form a shield over the nucleus of the living keratinocyte cells to prevent solar radiation damage. UV light also inflames the skin. The long-term effects of solar radiation cause pigment to pool from leaking melanocytes. This phenomenon produces age spots. In this case, the melanocyte has been damaged by UV exposure and needs to be repaired.

With injury or infection, a raised red breakout may form that eventually turns into a hyperpigmented spot because of an increase of melanin in the affected area. In a normal situation, when the redness subsides, the resulting hyperpigmentation simply falls off as the cell moves to the top of the epidermis.

SKIN LIGHTENING AGENTS

Hydroquinone

Tyrosinase is an enzyme that determines just how much melanin is produced. The majority of products available to treat hyperpigmentation inhibit tyrosinase in one way or another. Hydroquinone has been considered the gold standard for effective reduction of hyperpigmentation. It can be used to retard or stop production of melanin in many conditions, such as melasma or post-inflammatory hyperpigmentation. In rare cases, it may produce a progressive darkening of the area. Hydroquinone use should be discontinued if no improvements occur within four to six months. It is currently banned in Europe and some Asian countries. Pregnant women should not use it.

Most skin lightening ingredients work better as part of a combination than on their own. Skin brightening agents, such as kojic acid, are often combined with other ingredients such as azelaic acid, glycolic acids, lactic acid, retinol, ascorbic acid, and botanical lighteners for best results. The most effective hydroquinone combination that we have encountered is our privately compounded prescription strength lotion (B+Z clarifying lotion) containing hydroquinone, retinol, and a soothing chamomile extract.

Kojic Acid

Kojic acid comes from fungal and organic plant materials. It helps reduce melanin formation, and is similar to hydroquinone but can be less irritating to the skin. It scavenges free radicals that are released from cells and acts synergistically with magnesium ascorbyl phosphate to inhibit tyrosinase activity. Kojic acid, like hydroquinone, can also be combined with a variety of other ingredients to hasten improvement of pigment irregularities. We combine it with retinol and chamomile extract in our B+Z clarifying lotion for sensitive skin.

Glycolic Acid

The most common alpha hydroxy acids used in cosmeceutical formulations are glycolic acid and lactic acid. Glycolic acid is a wonderful base to apply before a bleaching agent because it helps draw the bleach into the skin by removing the top dead layer of epidermis. As part of our treatment protocol, we use weekly in-office glycolic acid peels and daily B+Z Smoothing Lotion at home to help hydroquinone and kojic acid penetrate and accelerate the pigment shedding process.

BV-OSC

BV-OSC is a highly stable derivative of ascorbic acid that demonstrates a longer time of effectiveness. It is an oil soluble esterified form of vitamin C, which makes it more stable and allows for improved skin penetration. It retains its potency longer than other forms of ascorbic acid that are delivered topically. A 10 percent concentration can suppress melanin formation and acts with kojic acid to inhibit tyrosinase activity. We have made this a component of Beautif-Eye™ Nourishing Cream.

OTHER INGREDIENTS THAT PROMOTE A MORE EVEN SKIN TONE

Our research to develop and perfect an eyelid product that reduces dark circles under the eyes as well as to "correct, protect and renew"™ eyelid skin—Beautifeye—has been very productive. We have incorporated exciting new ingredients that utilize new technologies that have never been available before—like Palmitoyl Tetrapeptide—and traditional Amazonian tribal remedies that we have never had access to before—Guarana, Cupuacu Butter, and Andiroba Oil.

Palmitoyl Tetrapeptide

Palmitoyl Tetrapeptide enhances the skin's capacity to eliminate the pigmented bi-products of hemoglobin. It increases eyelid skin density and supports the microvascular network around the eyes by combating vessel fragility.

Guarana

Guarana is a traditional Brazilian energizer that is often consumed instead of coffee and is considered a youth elixir. Research has found it to be a botanical cellular stimulator, enhancing cell turnover, increasing circulation, and reducing fatty deposits.

COMBINATION THERAPIES

Skin lightening is not a fast process. Depending upon how dark the area is, compared to your normal skin tone, it can take six months to see significant improvement.

Non-prescription lightening creams can go only so far in improving the appearance of melasma and dark circles.

If you want a more dramatic result, prescription strength lotions plus glycolic peels, trichloracetic acid (TCA) peels, microdermabrasion, and intense pulsed light (IPL) and photodynamic therapy (PDT) using Levulan™ treatments are recommended in multiple sessions.

Patients with darker skin types need a regimen to reduce post-inflammatory hyperpigmentation. Any treatment that creates irritation may cause the pigment to react. If your skin is prone to hyperpigmentation, a skin lightening and maintenance regimen should be followed on an ongoing basis to prevent pigmentary changes. You should also not be tanned at the time of an IPL or PDT treatment.

PEELING SOLUTIONS

Laser and other light sources have evolved rapidly, however, chemical peels are still an effective option to reverse the visible signs of sun-damaged skin and work hand in hand with newer technologies. The simplicity and affordability of chemical peels, unlike the higher cost of lasers, make peels a popular alternative for skin rejuvenation and maintenance. Working with our aestheticians, we offer a variety of choices to achieve the best results.

Chemical peeling began in ancient Egypt over 5000 years ago. Only fruit acids and lactic acids were then available. By the end of the nineteenth century, physicians started using salicylic acid, resorcinol, phenol, and trichloracetic acid. Phenol was first used to remove acne scars. The advent of alpha hydroxy acids and trichloracetic acid has made chemical peeling a safe and popular procedure.

Superficial peels treat fine wrinkles and dark spots, and acne. Usually we recommend starting with one peel a week for six weeks, and then a maintenance regimen of once a month is suggested, depending on the condition of your skin. Superficial glycolic peels require no recovery time and are safe for most skin types. Patients with rosacea or redness should be cautious since peels can increase the number of broken capillaries. Peels work best on women with pigment irregularities, blotches, fine wrinkles, open pores, and mild sun damage, and in combination with the other selections on the noninvasive facial rejuvenation menu—injectable therapies, intense pulsed light (IPL), photodynamic therapy, (PDT) and non-ablative lasers.

Medium depth peels are superb for improving moderately photodamaged skin when superficial glycolic acid peels just do not do enough. When the upper layer of your skin (stratum corneum) is thickened, cell turn over slows down and a build-up of debris causes a rough texture and a dull complexion. When the deeper layer of your skin (the dermis) suffers collagen and elastin degeneration, which appear as moderate to deep facial wrinkles, the results from medium depth (TCA) peels can be dramatic. But there are several days of recovery, which may not be acceptable to everyone.

Which peel is the best for me?

There are specific criteria we take into consideration when selecting a peeling agent.

CRITERIA
Fitzpatrick classification—skin type
Age
Lifestyle (sun exposure, alcohol, smoking)
Current skincare regimen
Previous skin treatments (peels, lasers, or other technology)
Facial cosmetic surgeries
Current medication, including Accutane®
Vitamin supplements
History of herpes simplex

Once your specific needs are understood, we can establish realistic expectations and healing times and make the best recommendation. Improvement will be cumulative and continue gradually over time. The results will be limited to the surface of the skin, the epidermis, and should be combined with a skincare regimen for optimal results.

Our philosophy is to look at skincare as a key part of a continuum—in office treatments combined with state-of-the-art cosmeceuticals. We recommend a pre-peel regimen that consists of lower concentration of alpha hydroxy acids, retinoids, bleaches, topical anti-oxidants, and sunscreen for at least two weeks prior to any peel treatment. A skin rejuvenation program takes a commitment of time, expense, discipline, and most importantly, sun avoidance and protection. If you are not willing to make the necessary lifestyle changes required, do not start a peel program.

THE ART OF THE PEEL

Superficial Peels: Alpha Hydroxy Acid Peels

Alpha hydroxy acids (AHA) treat fine wrinkling, hyperpigmentation, melasma, and acne. Glycolic acid creates a thinning of the outer layer of the skin, improving the texture and uniformity of the skin and allowing other topical agents to work better. As a peeling agent, glycolic acid may be used in concentrations of 30 to 50 percent (by aestheticians) and 50 to 70 percent (by physicians). Glycolic acids have to be neutralized either by rinsing it off with water or by applying a neutralizing solution to turn them off, in effect. Factors affecting the depth of penetration of a glycolic peel are the concentration, method of application, skin pre-treatment, and duration of the acid in contact with the skin. After cleaning your face, we apply the peel, leaving it on for a maximum of ten minutes. We neutralize the peel as soon as we see you becoming slightly pink.

POST AHA PEEL CARE: A mild moisturizer is used three times a day for two days. If there is any redness, we recommend a mild topical steroid cream. After any inflammation is gone, you can resume using alpha hydroxy acids and retinoids.

The neck, chest, and the back of the hands—areas that we do not treat with ablative lasers—are also effectively treated with AHA peels and photodynamic therapy.

AVOIDING POTENTIAL COMPLICATIONS (THESE RULES APPLY TO ALL PEELS)

- **HERPES**—if you have a history of cold sores, you should take antiviral medication before and after your peel

- **REDNESS**—may be treated with mild topical steroid creams

- **INFECTION & SCARRING**—very rare

A light AHA peel can be repeated on a weekly basis to achieve glowing skin without any downtime. We begin with low concentrations and gradually increase the strength of the peel with each successive treatment.

Medium Depth Peels: TCA Peels (Trichloracetic Acid Peels)

TCA peels can range from superficial to medium depth depending on the concentration. Concentrations of 10 to 20 percent are primarily exfoliants and affect the outside layer of the epidermis. We recommend these for mild signs of sun damage of the face, neck, and chest.

TCA peels in concentrations from 30 percent to 40 percent are considered medium depth peels. The concentration is the most important factor that determines the depth of the peel, however, other factors such as skin type, skin preparation, number of layers applied, and the method of application, also influence the depth of the peel.

STEPS FOR A TCA PEEL

- **SKIN PREPARATION**—The skin is primed with alpha hydroxy acids, retinoids, and bleaching agents two weeks prior to the peel

- **CLEANSING**—A thorough cleansing to eliminate debris with a toner and degreasing the skin with alcohol or acetone is performed

- **APPLICATION**—The depth of the peel is increased with each additional layer that is applied. We extend the peel into the hairline and just below the jawline to avoid a very visible demarcation line.

- **FROSTING**—Once the peel is applied we wait for it to frost. It does not have to be neutralized like glycolic acid does. There is a burning sensation that lasts several minutes, but we apply soothing cold compresses.

- **POST PEEL CARE**—A gentle cleanser and moisturizer are required during the four to five days following the peel. You will resume your normal skincare routine with Retin-A®, alpha hydroxy acids and sun block in 7-10 days.

Medium depth peels require a slightly longer time for healing. Initially the skin will have a leathery appearance, and it will turn from light to dark brown within 72 hours. Flaking may occur on areas with more muscular activity (around eyes, mouth, and forehead). Patients wash their face with a gentle cleanser and apply only petrolatum-based formulas and antibiotic ointment, and a mild hydrocortisone to reduce itching.

POST PEEL RULES

- Avoid sun during the healing period
- Avoid picking the skin ; do not remove any of the brown crust by picking
- Try to sleep on your back as much as possible.
- A prophylactic antiviral medication will be prescribed if you have history of cold sores.

MICRODERMABRASION

Microdermabrasion is a popular mechanical alternative to light chemical peels.

Through a wand-like hand piece, tiny sterile aluminum oxide or salt crystals are delivered at a high velocity onto the skin's surface and immediately vacuumed away, taking the top-most layer of dead skin cells with it. It is usually performed on the face and neck, but can also be performed on the hands, chest, arms, and legs. A new technique Aqua-abrasion uses suction and water under pressure. It is less traumatic to the skin and does not involve the use of crystals.

Microdermabrasion is used to improve rough skin texture, mild scarring, uneven pigmentation, and superficial brown spots. It is also useful for acne lesions, blackheads, and fine wrinkles. One of its main advantages is that it can be safely used on all skin types. A typical regimen consists of a series of four to eight treatments done at intervals of two to four weeks. Immediately after the procedure, the skin has a pink glow and makeup can be applied.

We use microdermabrasion on the outer layer of the skin, which signals the lower layers of the epidermis to produce new skin cells and stimulates the dermis to increase production of elastin and collagen. It is a very versatile procedure and can be combined with other techniques such as glycolic peels and intense pulsed light therapy. Using microdermabrasion before a peel will allow the peel to penetrate more deeply. Using microdermabrasion after IPL will speed up the fading of pigmented spots.

MICRODERMABRASION VS PEELS VS LASERS (each method removes the most superficial layers of the skin)	
MICRODERMABRASION	*Mechanical*
PEELS	*Chemical*
LASERS	*Thermal*

CHAPTER 12

Using Dermal Fillers to Restore Facial Contours

In the 1980's, we started with bovine collagen, and now the category of dermal fillers has evolved into a maintstay of cosmetic medicine with a widening selection of materials.

This chapter will bring you up to date on the newest developments with filling agents from all over the world.

Now we have a broad spectrum of safe and reliable materials that are readily available and that fit in well with our concept of combination therapies. We use them in combination with Botox®, non-ablative and ablative lasers, IPL (intense pulsed light), LED therapies, and Thermage®.

THE PERFECT FILLER

When it comes to long-lasting fillers, forever would be preferable if we did not have to sacrifice safety for longevity.

Patients and doctors want a wrinkle filler that can be administered safely, conveniently, rapidly, painlessly, and without traces that it has been used. We want a product that does not result in any complications and that lasts a long time.

For years bovine collagen was the only legally available filling material. Since many patients were allergic to it (it is a product taken from cows), it required two skin tests, a month apart, to test for allergies. As imperfect as it was, it was a beginning. Silicone was used by some physicians. Although it is chemically inert, the silicone used in the past was often not standardized and contained impurities that produced severe reactions. Silicone is permanent. Unfortunately when it was injected in large qualtities it often migrated and was difficult or impossible to remove. More refined, highly purified silicone, silicone that is used intraocularly for correction of detached retinas, is now available.

When it is injected with a microdroplet technique, the complications can be minimized and the results satisfactory, but its uses are limited.

We have not yet achieved the ideal filler, but the non-animal-derived stabilized hyaluronic acid products opened the door to the current state of the art, fulfilling much of our desired criteria. Each filler that we use has its own indications and attributes. We can map out the face, using different fillers in different areas (see Figures 3 and 4).

FILLER INDICATIONS

FOREHEAD FURROWS	Restylane®, Hylaform®, Captique™
TEMPLE DEPRESSIONS & FLATTENING	Sculptra®, Perlane®
GLABELLA, "YOUR 11"	Restylane®, Perlane®, Hylaform®, Hylaform® Plus
LOWER EYELID DEPRESSIONS, TEAR TROUGH DEFORMITIES	Restylane®, Perlane®, Hylaform®, Hylaform® Plus
NASOLABIAL FOLDS	Restylane®, Perlane®, Radiesse™, Hylaform®, Hylaform® Plus
CHEEKBONES	Sculptra®, Radiesse™
CHEEK DEPRESSIONS	Sculptra®
MARIONETTE LINES	Restylane®, Perlane®, Sculptra®, Hylaform®, Hylaform® Plus
UPPER LIP LINES	Restylane®, Restylane® Touch, Captique™, Cosmoderm®, Cosmoplast®

UPPER & LOWER LIP BORDERS	Restylane®, Cosmoderm®, Cosmoplast®
BODY OF LIP	Restylane Lipp®, Perlane®, Hylaform®, Hylaform® Plus
JOWLS	Perlane®, Radiesse™, Sculptra®
NOSE	Restylane®, Perlane®, Radiesse™
CHIN	Radiesse™
NECK	Restylane® Vital

STATIC WRINKLES

Wrinkles, grooves, creases, furrows, and fine lines that are the result of aging, sun exposure, and loss of elasticity can be filled to create a smoother surface and the illusion of a more youthful face. Facial animation (squinting, smoking) and a variety of facial expressions (smiling, frowning, crying, and being surprised) accentuate wrinkles in areas of the face. The muscles causing these dynamic wrinkles have to be relaxed with Botox® to get the best results with fillers.

While theoretically any facial area can be filled, some areas typically require a different material than others. For instance, using a filler to reinflate sunken cheeks will have to be different than the filler used to camouflage your lower lid bags.

Where to avoid fillers

There are some facial areas that we do not usually recommend filling. For example, we do not usually recommend filling crow's feet creases unless the lines are exceptionally deep. The skin is too fine and the muscle activity too rapid and repetitive in the crow's feet area. These lines are much more efficiently managed with botulinum toxin.

Fillers Around the Eyes

We use fillers around the eye area and to camouflage lower lid bags and indentations. The procedure has to be performed very meticulously because eyelid skin, especially in women, is very delicate and often translucent. Hyaluronic acid fillers—which are the safest material to be injected around the eye—may show through the thin skin and look gray. So the filler has to be placed under the muscle instead of under the skin. We have described a technique called the Restylane® Push to fill in depressions near the nose—tear trough deformity—or when a patient has had too much fat removed during an eyelift. In some patients, filling in these depressions can also improve the appearance of lower lid bags by filling in the shadow under your lower lid bags if you are not emotionally ready for a surgical procedure.

The Nasolabial Folds

Nasolabial folds—the grooves along side of your nose—are prime regions for filling to camouflage mid-facial laxity. Sometimes these folds get deeper as the result of facial deflating, like the wrinkles in a balloon as the air is let out of it. We use a combination of different fillers in different facial areas to get the desired result. First we reinflate the cheeks with Sculptra®, then we fill the nasolabial folds with a layering of thicker and thinner materials for an enhanced effect. The deep layers can be filled with Perlane® or Radiesse™. This can even elevate the midfacial area as well as filling in the groove. The finer, more superficial lines can be filled with Restylane® or Hylaform®. The results can be further enhanced with skin tightening procedures like Thermage® or augmentation of the cheek bones with Sculptra® or Radiesse™. Following mid-face lifting or tightening procedures, using filling agents in the nasolabial grooves may be necessary to get the final effect that you want.

Marionette Lines

Marionette lines—those grooves that begin at the corners of your mouth and continue down to your chin—are effectively treated with filling agents. But when the lines are deep and the corners of the mouth point downward, we need Botox® to relax the muscles that are pulling the mouth down and we need Thermage® to lift and tighten the midface, in addition to the use of fillers, to give a more complete correction.

We have devised a technique of layering thicker more deeply injected fillers and more superficially injected thinner fillers for a smoother effect. We also use this combination technique of layered fillers to support the downturned corners of the mouth. We support the corners of the mouth and the outside corners of the upper and lower lips with thicker fillers. We use Perlane® for the corners of the mouth and we use Sculptra® for the marionette area below the corners of the mouth.

Using fillers artfully is all about having a keen aesthetic eye, layering and knowing what to use where.

Facial Recontouring and Restylane® Rhinoplasty

Recontouring of the facial bony contours (cheek bones, chin, jawline) can be achieved with thicker fillers (Perlane®, Sculptra®, Radiesse™) injected more deeply under the muscle, rather then just under the skin. This will give you immediate gratification and a chance to have enhanced facial contour without surgery. We have been performing Restylane® rhinoplasty to correct nasal asymmetries for several years with great success on patients who have had multiple surgical procedures and are no longer surgical candidates.

Other Uses for Fillers

Small traumatic and pitted acne scars can be filled with droplets of Restylane® or silicone. It usually takes multiple sessions to correct depressions from scar tissue. Each injection will release some of the scar tissue, allowing more to be injected at the next visit. We have even used Restylane® and Perlane® during surgery to keep new scar tissue from forming and keeping tissue in the right place. Broad areas of scarring or facial atrophy require thicker materials and larger volumes (fat, Sculptra®, Radiesse™).

FILLER CHOICES

We have worked with many filling materials in Europe and South America before they were available in the US, and have shared the clinical insights of our colleagues from around the world. We have had the opportunity to preview their potential uses and complications. Based on these experiences, we have decided which products would be the safest and most effective to use for our patients.

Filling agents can be derived from natural materials (like hyaluronic acid that is present in every living organism) or from synthetic materials (like poly lactic acid that is in Sculptra®). They can be derived from animals (Hylaform® is from roosters, bovine collagen comes from cows); from human tissue (Cosmoderm® and Cosmoplast®); and from your own tissue (Isolagen).

Filling agents fill. They can fill in lines and furrows and depressions. They can also be volumizers that reinflate deflated tissue and plump up broad areas.

Fillers have an immediate effect. You will see improvement before you leave the office. There may be some swelling which accentuates the effect of the filler, but this is usually gone within a day or so. You may think that the filler in your lip has disappeared when your lips look slightly smaller several days after your treatment. We tell our patients that if they like the size of their lips on the day following a lip augmentation, they will probably want more. The effects of some temporary fillers, like Sculptra®, improve over several months, but eventually they will diminish with time. Depending on which filler is used on which part of the face, it can last from three months to two years.

Dangers of Permanent Fillers

In general we do not recommend permanent fillers. We use purified silicone (Silikon 1000) very sparingly, in microdroplets, to correct depressed facial scars. There are several permanent injectable products, containing synthetic materials and polymethyl methacrylate beads suspended in collagen, that are being used in Europe and Canada (including ArteFill®, DermaLive®, DermaDeep®). We will not use these materials because there have been serious complications reported.

The general rule is that permanent fillers can cause permanent complications.

HYALURONIC ACID

Because we have had so many years of experience with hyaluronic acid and have seen how safe and effective it is, this has been our preferred filling material since 1995. This substance is one of the pillars of our non-invasive facial rejuvenation technique.

Hyaluronic acid is a polysaccharide that is in all tissues; each of us has hyaluronic acid in all of the organs in our bodies. The largest amount of hyaluronic acid in our bodies is in our skin. Patients often call these fillers "sugar gels" since polysaccharides are chemically related to sugars. Because hyaluronic acid has a simple chemical structure that is identical in all species and tissues, it is an ideal filling material. When the body breaks down hyaluronic acid, it becomes carbon dioxide and water, and leaves no foreign material in your body. These products produce longer lasting results and fewer allergic reactions than collagen products.

Hyaluronic acid derived from rooster combs has been

used for almost three decades by ophthalmic surgeons during intraocular surgical procedures. This intraocular hyaluronic acid was cross-linked—connected to other molecules—to make it thicker and to last longer. We were the first to use this new crosslinked product to reconstruct monkey eyelids, eye globes, and eye sockets (1990–1995), and we were among a few selected physicians who participated in its early development to enhance and replace volume in the reconstructive and cosmetic arenas. A variation of this product later became marketed as Hylaform®.

A non-animal derived form of hyaluronic acid became available several years later. Restylane®, a non-animal stabilized hyaluronic acid (NASHA) is produced by Q-Med AB, Uppsala, Sweden. It is made by fermentation using bacteria and is not derived from an animal source. We have used Restylane® extensively since 1996 for adding volume to facial structures and for softening lines and folds.

We instruct our patients that if the correction that they see is less apparent in five to seven days, this is not because the gel has dissipated, but because they need more volume implanted. We ask our patients to return in seven to ten days for a possible touch-up. Skin testing before injection is not necessary with hyaluronic acid products. Some doctors report that they see more bruising and swelling with hyaluronic acid fillers. We have not seen this. And we have not seen any localized inflammatory reactions since 1996 when the hyaluronic acid purification process was improved. We have documented our findings in over 2,400 patients in an article published in the Archives of Facial Plastic Surgery (November, 2004).

Because hyaluronic acid gel products offer reproducible results, they are readily accepted by doctors and patients alike and are very popular. The difference between the different hyaluronic acid products is the amount of hyaluronic acid that each contains, the origin of the hyaluronic acid (animal or non-animal) and the amount and nature of its chemical crosslinking. The Q-Med hyaluronic acid products contain 20mg/ml of hyaluronic acid, while Hylaform® and Captique™ contain 5.5 mg/ml of hyaluronic acid. Q-med has patented the amount and the nature of the crosslinking in Restylane®. There is enough to make Restylane® last longer, but not too much to limit the amount of water that it can absorb. The more water that the hyaluronic acid molecule can absorb, the more volume it can maintain for a longer period of time. This explains why Restylane® lasts longer than Hylaform® and Captique™, and why Perlane® lasts longer than Hylaform® Plus.

In 2005 Hylaform® Plus (a thicker version of Hylaform®) and Captique™ (a non-animal version of Hylaform®) were FDA approved. Awaiting approval are Juvéderm® (Inamed, rooster derived homogenous hyaluronic acid gel that reportedly is easier to inject) and Perlane® (the thicker version of Restylane®).

THE EUROPEAN EXPERIENCE

In Europe there are many new hyaluronic acid products:

• Visagel® (heavily crossed homogenous non-animal hyaluronic acid gel)

• Hydrafil® (non-animal homogenous hyaluronic acid gel)

• Softline® (non-animal crosslinked hyaluronic acid suspended in non-crosslinked hyaluronic acid)

• Softline® Max (non-animal crosslinked hyaluronic acid)

• Puragen® (rooster derived double crosslinked hyaluronic acid)

• Belotero® (rooster derived crosslinked hyaluronic acid in a "soft gel")

• Restylane Lipp® – intermediate thickness (between Restylane and Perlane)

• Restylane® Vital – not crosslinked – "softer" (easily massaged into tissue for skin plumping rather than filling)

Crosslinked fillers last longer, but are more rigid (more difficult to inject and more difficult to mold). The non-crosslinked hyaluronic acid fillers are more flexible. The homogenous hyaluronic acid gels have better flow characteristics (easier to inject).

PRODUCT	DURATION OF EFFECT	FDA APPROVAL	FORMULATION
RESTYLANE® MEDICIS, SCOTTSDALE, AZ	6-9 Months	FDA approved December 12, 2003	Has 20mg/ml of hyaluronic acid with a gel bead size of 250 micrometers and 100,000 units per ml
HYLAFORM® ALLERGAN	4-5 Months	FDA approved 2004	5.5mg/ml hyaluronic acid
CAPTIQUE® ALLERGAN	4-5 Months	FDA approved 2004	5.5mg/ml hyaluronic acid
PERLANE® Q-MED, UPPSALA, SWEDEN	9-12 Months	Not approved yet in the United States	Has 20mg/ml of hyaluronic acid with a gel bead size of 1000 micrometers and 10,000 units per ml
HYLAFORM PLUS® ALLERGAN	6-8 Months	FDA approved 2005	5.5 mg/ml hyaluronic acid
RESTYLANE® FINE LINES Q-MED UPPSALA, SWEDEN	3-6 Months	Not approved yet in the United States	Has 20mg/ml of hyaluronic acid with a gel bead size of 100 micrometers and 250,000 units per ml

The duration of non-animal derived hyaluronic is dependent on the size of the gel particle and its concentration. Hyaluronic acid attracts and holds water, that is how it maintains its volume and plumps up tissue.

We have used Restylane® for superficial lines and moderate wrinkles and furrows with great success since 1996. We inject it into the middle layer of the skin, not too superficially so that the clear gel does not show through the skin and appears gray. The effects last an average of nine months; the glabellar creases and nasolabial fold corrections last longer than lip body and marionette line corrections. After about six months some of the lines and furrows may start to reappear, but at least half of the Restylane® will still be in the tissue where it was injected. This material, still in place at the previous injection sites, acts as a foundation for subsequent injections. Thus new injections of Restylane® will add to the effect of the previous injections. These secondary injections provide enhanced and longer-lasting corrections. This same concept works for layering Restylane® on a foundation of deeper, thicker Perlane®.

Will lip enhancing products (like gels and glosses) prolong the effects of Restylane®?

Yes, any over the counter lip enhancing product will cause some swelling. Since Restylane® attracts water, the use of the two together will have a more profound effect.

We have used Perlane®, although it is not yet available in the United States, with great success in Europe and South America since 2000 to fill in deep facial furrows and contour irregularities. Because it is thicker, it will last longer than Restylane®. Restylane® can be layered over a foundation of Perlane® for correction of residual superficial irregularities. Perlane® is injected more deeply into the skin or it can be injected under the skin as well.

We have used Restylane® Fine Lines (Restylane® Touch,

not available in the United States) since 2000 for correction of delicate upper lip wrinkles. Because it is used in smaller quantities, it has a shorter duration, averaging three to four months. Captique®, Cosmoderm®, and Cosmoplast® are also useful filler materials for softening upper lip lines and accentuating the borders of the lips.

Hylaform® and Hylaform® Plus, are also clear, colorless, transparent gel implants composed of crosslinked molecules of hyaluronic acid, but they are extracted from minced rooster combs and may contain avian protein, which may subject them to a higher level of impurities or contaminants. Hylaform® (less viscous) is used in similar fashion to Restylane® and Hylaform® Plus (more viscous) is used in a similar fashion to Perlane®. Perlane® has larger hyaluronic acid bead sizes and Hylaform® Plus has more crosslinking, which theoretically may prevent it from attracting enough water to produce as long lasting an effect as Perlane®.

Hyaluronic acid products do not contain any anesthetic agent. To make you more comfortable during the injections, we apply Photocaine™ topical anesthetic in a thick layer fifteen to thirty minutes before your injections. This is a privately compounded product that works better than most commercially available numbing creams and will make your experience more pleasant. After injection, gentle massage helps to achieve a smooth and continuous contour with the surrounding tissue and decreases the chance of brusing. Taking three Arnica Montana 6X pellets under your tongue every two hours following your injection will also decrease your chances of bruising.

Captique™ (Allergan)

Captique™ is basically the same as Hylaform® with the major difference that it is made by bacterial fermentation rather than harvested from rooster combs. Aside from making the roosters happy, this allows the product to be produced without any animal proteins that theoretically can cause allergic reactions. It is the same concentration and thickness as

Hylaform®. We have found that it lasts as long as Hylaform®, but not as long as Restylane®.

Juvéderm® (Allergan)

Juvéderm® is a slightly different hyaluronic acid fillers. It is a homogenous gel that does not contain gel particles like Restylane® and so has better flow characteristics. It is rooster derived. Three versions are presently available that vary in concentration, and are well suited to a broad range of applications ranging from filling fine lines with a less dense product—Juvéderm® 18—to softening deep nasolabial furrows with a more dense one such as Juvéderm® 30. Lips may be plumped with Juvéderm® 24. Juvéderm® has recently been approved by the FDA.

POLYLACTIC ACID

We are using this product more and more because it has a specific use and is complementary to our use of hyaluronic acid. It is FDA approved for the correction of HIV related facial muscle wasting (myodystrophy). Sculptra® (Dermik Laboratories) was originally called Newfill® when we used it in Europe and South America. It is a suspension of microparticles of synthetic poly-L-lactic acid (the same material used in absorbable sutures) that has to be mixed with sterile water. Right before it is injected, xylocaine (a local anesthetic) is added to the suspension. Sculptra® is a volumizer, and not a wrinkle filler. It reinflates facial areas that have become deflated. Rather than filling in specific lines, wrinkles, or folds, it plumps up large areas, making wrinkles disappear and giving a full, youthful appearance. We have found that this product works well to fill in broad irregular areas. Because the amount of correction improves with time, inciting a mild subcutaneous inflammatory response and secondary collagen production, we prefer a gradual filling in of contour defects at one to two month intervals. The ultimate result may last up to two years.

To avoid lumps or inflammation around injected material,

we mix the power in a larger volume of sterile water, inject
very small amounts in many locations, inject deeply under
the skin, and massage the injection sites.

HYDROXYLAPATITE

Radiesse™ (Bioform, Franksville, Wisconsin) is tiny spherical
particles of synthetic hydroxylapatite crystals blended in a
gel containing water, glycerin, and carboxymethylcellulose.
It is FDA approved for use in the vocal cords, radiological
soft tissue marking, and for dental and maxillofacial bone
grafting. Hydroxylapatite is a component of bone and teeth.
In this product it is used to stimulate new collagen formation rather than to stimulate bone growth. Because of this
bony component, we have hesitated to use it within the skin
as a wrinkle filler, but it has some advantages as a volumizer
to recontour bony facial prominences, and as a subcutaneous support for the midface and around the mouth. We have
found it most useful to accentuate cheek bones and chins,
injecting it under muscle and layering it over the bone. It can
also be used to fill in very deep nasolabial folds and marionette lines. Results can last one to two years.

Collagen

**Approximately 25 percent of the protein in the human body
and 75 percent in the skin is collagen.**

For the last three decades, the most widely available and
widely used substance for filling in facial lines has been
bovine collagen. It requires skin testing at four and again
at eight weeks to identify patients with sensitivity to the
implant because it is from animal sources. Even patients with
two negative skin tests may have a reaction. If you have had
an allergic reaction to bovine collagen in the past, you may
also be allergic to human collagen products (Cosmoderm®
and Cosmoplast®).

Although we have never offered bovine collagen products in our practices, many patients who have used them for years were satisfied with their results. The average longevity of correction with these products is about three months. It can be used in combination with hyaluronic acid fillers.

Zyderm® 1 is highly purified bovine dermal collagen. Zyderm® 2 is a slightly thicker form of bovine collagen. Both contain 0.3 percent lidocaine to provide local anesthesia on injection. The FDA approved Zyderm® 1 in 1981 and Zyderm® 2 was approved in 1983. Zyplast® is used for correction of deeper skin wrinkles and the results last longer than Zyderm®. The FDA approved it in 1985.

CosmoDerm® is purified collagen from human fibroblast cell culture that is grown under controlled conditions. It contains 0.3 percent lidocaine as local anesthetic. This is the second generation of injectable collagen fillers, approved by the FDA in 2003. CosmoDerm® 1 and CosmoDerm® 2 have the same indications as their predecessors—Zyderm® 1 and Zyderm® 2. CosmoPlast® is recommended for the correction of deeper folds such as nasolabial folds and marionette lines. The persistence of results using these products is comparable to the bovine-derived products.

Because of the flow characteristics and lidocaine content of the CosmoDerm® and CosmoPlast®, there are some practical advantages to using these products in combination with hyaluronic acid products. For instance, using CosmoPlast® to first outline upper lip borders, will numb the lip and facilitate augmentation of the body of the lip with Restylane® or Perlane®.

ISOLAGEN

Isolagen is a process whereby a patient's own cells are extracted, reproduced, and then reintroduced. The Isolagen process utilizes only the patient's unique, living cells to produce the patient's own collagen. There is no foreign substance used. Isolagen's approach is different from other temporary injectable fillers (except for fat) because it uses your own fibroblasts to create more collagen, which is then injected into the areas of your face where you need it. The use of autologous cellular therapies has the potential to avoid many of the complications of introducing foreign substances into your skin. We have found that it is an expensive and time consuming process (your cells need weeks to be grown in the lab), and does not give the immediate gratification that most fillers give. At the present time, it is awaiting FDA approval in the US but is available in Europe.

AUTOLOGOUS FAT

In theory, the idea of taking fat from where you do not want it and putting it where you need it is very appealing.

Using autologous material—tissue from your own body—has always been our preferred method for reconstructing eyelids. If you use your own tissue, then your body cannot reject it and it can give a permanent result. The use of your own fat as a filling agent has the advantages of potential permanence after implantation and there is unlimited volume available for implantation. We can all find some site on our bodies where we can harvest fat. Some fat cells may also become stem cells and will rejuvenate the skin and subcutaneous facial structures as well.

This technique has the disadvantage of requiring an additional procedure for harvesting, and there can be an extended period of swelling after the procedure that can last for several weeks. When fat transplantation is performed in an artful manner, the results can be gratifying. However, especially around the eyelids, there can be areas where the fat survives and other areas where it does not, leaving lumps that are difficult to remove. In this era of immediate gratification without downtime, autologous fat transplantation is not for every patient.

OTHER HUMAN TISSUE IMPLANTS

Other non-autologous (from humans, but not your own tissue) materials have been used as fillers. We have not found them useful and do not use them because they cause more swelling than the hyaluronic acid fillers and do not last. Alloderm® is a solid acellular biological implant that has been used for repairing large facial contour deformities. Human dermal tissue is harvested from cadavers. The cells are removed without altering the collagen and cell structure of the skin. The resulting skin serves as a framework to support revascularization and cellular repopulation. Cymetra® is a micronized, injectable form of Alloderm®. When it is injected for lip augmentation, we have commonly seen considerable swelling and rapid resorption.

PERMANENT FILLERS

The search for permanent synthetic fillers has been fraught with controversy worldwide. Materials that appear to give satisfying results in the short term, may ultimately lead to complications after several years. With the exception of the silicone microdroplet technique, which can be useful when used in small quantities, at this time we do not use permanent filling agents because they cannot be removed easily. Although there is improvement in the development of solid implants for the lips, we still do not use them because of their tendency to extrude and the visibility of their edges.

INJECTABLE SILICONE

Silicone is a permanent filler that has been used since the 1940's. However, it has been misused during the subsequent decades. Excessive volumes and non-medical grade forms have caused subsequent complications and controversy. Two FDA-approved medical-grade liquid injectable silicones are available today. Adatosil® (Escalon Medical Corp. Chicago, Il) and Silikon® (Alcon Laboratories, Fort Worth, TX) are approved for the tamponade of retinal detachments. The FDA's Modernization Act (1997) allows for their off-label use for soft tissue augmentation.

Microdroplet, serial puncture technique is the safest and most efficacious use of liquid silicone. The goal of this technique is to undercorrect initially, using small volume injections and at each subsequent treatment session, at one to three month intervals, until the desired result is obtained. Silicone can create problems if too much is injected. Larger volumes can migrate with time and because of the adjacent inflammatory reaction, these masses of silicone will be difficult or impossible to remove, leaving significant soft tissue deformities. We have seen patients who have had large volumes of silicone injected into their cheek bone twenty years ago and now have massive deformities of their jowls—where the silicone migrated.

COMPLICATIONS & RISKS OF PERMANENT FILL

• Hardening and lumps	• Migration
• Chronic inflammation	• Infections
• Rashes	• Allergic reactions
• Extrusion	• Acne pustules

FILLER TECHNIQUES

We follow a specific regimen before each dermal filler treatment to make the experience pleasant. The use of Arnica Montana decreases the chance of bruising and minimizes swelling. We give our patients three sublingual Arnica 6X pellets before or immediately after their treatment and ask them to continue taking them four times daily for three days (or longer if you get bruising).

We use our specially compounded topical anesthetic cream, and rarely find it necessary to use regional nerve blocks or dental blocks, even for lip augmentation. The longer we leave the topical anesthetic in place, the better it works.

Men are much less tolerant of discomfort than women, but even men do not mind these treatments after we have used our specially compounded numbing cream for thirty minutes or more (women only require fifteen minutes).

How long do they last?

Each temporary filler has an inherent breakdown time or longevity. The greater the volume used and the less mobile the tissue into which it is implanted, the longer it will last. Complementary therapies such as botulinum toxin treatments and Thermage® will increase the persistence of the desired filling effect. Filling glabellar furrows (your "11") with Restylane® after the muscles have been relaxed with Botox® can yield satisfactory smoothing of the glabellar for nine to twelve months. About 20 percent of our patients who have been treated in this area with the combination of Botox® and Restylane® can be maintained with Botox® and do not need to be filled again. Other skin therapies, while they may not increase the longevity, will certainly improve the results. Chemical peels, IPL, PDT and non-ablative lasers will improve skin texture and thus make the effects of filling appear even better.

HOW LONG DO OUR MOST OFTEN USED FILLERS LAST?	
COSMODERM® **& COSMOPLAST®** (HUMAN DERIVED COLLAGEN)	Last an average of two to three months, slightly less than bovine collagen
RESTYLANE® (NON-ANIMAL DERIVED HYALURONIC ACID)	Lasts an average of six months (the nasolabial furrows lasting slightly longer while the area around the lips slightly less). Lasts longer than Hylaform®, Captique™, and Juvéderm® 18

PERLANE® (NON-ANIMAL DERIVED HYALURONIC ACID) — THICKER FORM	Lasts an average of nine months. Lasts longer than Hylaform® Plus and Juvéderm® 24
RADIESSE™ (HYDROXYLAPATITE SUSPENSION)	Lasts one to two years
SCULPTRA® (POLY LACTIC ACID)	May last for two years after being applied in a series of treatments over several months to achieve the final result

Can there be side effects?

Localized bruising can be minimized with the use of Arnica Montana before and after treatment, topical anesthetic agents that constrict blood vessels, cooling with masks and ice before and after the injections, and the application of pressure directly over the injection sites. Based on our experiences in Europe and South America, we avoid products and techniques that can cause lumps, granulomas, or skin reactions, including bovine collagen, or products that contain polymethylmethacrylate (PMMA) microspheres or polyacrylamide gel.

High patient satisfaction

In the November 2004 Archives of Facial Plastic Surgery, we reported on our six-year experience using Restylane® in more than 1,400 consecutive patients in our Dr Zilkha's oculoplastic clinic in Rio de Janeiro, Brazil. Patient satisfaction and durability of the procedures were evaluated at three, six, and nine months. For all treatment areas combined, at three months 88 percent of patients said they were satisfied or very satisfied with the procedure. The satisfaction rate for treatment areas combined was 73 percent at six months and 61 percent at nine months. But there were some facial areas where the satisfaction rate was much higher. The areas with both the most durable results and the highest patient satisfaction were the glabellar area and the nasolabial folds, where more than 80 percent of patients were still happy with the results at nine months. Patient satisfaction was highest for lip and marionette furrow procedures during the first three months, but the results did not last as long as in other areas. At these two sites, touch-ups were needed by six months. Patients who had injections into the glabellar area had been pretreated with Botox® to relax the corrugator muscles (which create the vertical lines between the eyebrows) and the procerus muscle (which creates horizontal furrows on the bridge of the nose). The Botox® relaxed the muscles and then any residual furrows were filled in. By using both, we can get a result that lasts much longer than by using either one by itself. About 20 percent of patients who had the two techniques together did not need the filler again and were maintained with only a couple of Botox® injections a year.

FILLERS OF THE FUTURE

New injectable tissue augmentation materials are constantly under development. Restylane® Sub Q is three times more viscous and longer lasting than Perlane®, lasting approximately one year. It is implanted with a cannula just above bone in areas where we want to accentuate bony prominences. In Sweden, Q-med is also working on Macrolane®, which is even more viscous and lasts for about two years and is undergoing clinical trials as an injectable breast implant. There are also many new hyaluronic acid fillers on the way from Europe and Asia.

We look forward to fillers of the future that will not cause any allergic reactions, will be long lasting, and will stimulate continuing rejuvenation of the skin, subcutaneous fat, and supportive facial tissues. In the future the use of stem cells may fulfill these ideals, plumping up the face and rejuvenating the skin.

CHAPTER 13

Acquiring an Ageless Smile

There are two key barometers of facial expression that are under constant assessment during most visible communication between people: the area around the eyes and the area around the mouth.

The periorbital and perioral areas serve as barometers send messages of openness or rejection, receptiveness or hostility, pleasure or pain, sadness or joy, understanding or misunderstanding, comprehension or confusion, and delight or despair.

Unfortunately, the dynamics of aging may create anatomical contours that sometimes send misleading messages about what is being sent and received. The result is a misinterpretation of attitude and response. For example, the thin lips of aging may suggest mean spiritedness. The downturn at the angles of the mouth suggests displeasure, grumpiness, or even anger. Thin wrinkled lips suggest old age and sub-optimal health. A weak chin-jaw complex usually results in a double chin and a square face, suggesting chubbiness even if you are trim. The deficient chin conveys a suggestion of weak personality or character. Of course, this has no relationship to reality, but people with strong chins and good jaw lines, up-turned corners of their mouths, and full lips may be perceived as more desirable.

Rejuvenation of this area can make a significant impact, but treating this area requires planning and the use of combination therapies. Rejuvenation of the perioral area needs more than soft tissue augmentation and muscle balance adjustment. The first step is often adjustment and alignment of your teeth and the restoration of your dental volume. This will establish dental support for the perioral area and create the foundation for our use of non-invasive combination therapies.

Loss of midfacial bony volume accentuates perioral aging changes. Our preliminary findings in an ongoing study using Radiesse™ to restore midfacial bony volume and support the midfacial area are giving us encouragement that this technique could be helpful.

Once the midfacial volume loss has been corrected or compensated for, then we can proceed with adjusting perioral muscle balance and fill in contour irregularities and any residual volume deficiency. We can define and enhance lip borders and contours with fillers and micropigmentation and we can augment lip volume with additional filler materials.

Artistically created micropigmentation is critical to the full rejuvenation of the perioral area. It replaces lip border pigment that has been lost with age and sun exposure. It redefines lip contour asymmetries and optically enhances lip volume. With the addition of a new lip border, volume augmentation of the body of the lip is not necessary as frequently.

THE FIVE-STEP APPROACH TO PERIORAL REJUVENATION

STEP ONE	Compensation for midfacial bone volume loss
STEP TWO	Establishment of dental support
STEP THREE	Botox® plus soft tissue filling
STEP FOUR	Laser resurfacing of the upper lip skin (when indicated)
STEP FIVE	Augmentation and micropigmentation of the lips

After the reestablishment of midfacial volume and dental contours, the soft tissue around the mouth can be addressed. Botox® sets the stage and prolongs the results of effective filling. Placement of the injection sites and dosages must be precise to avoid any imbalance of mouth movements. We use two units to each muscle to subtly elevate the corners of the mouth and soften marionette lines, and to facilitate filling of this area. The corners of the mouth and the outside corners of the upper and lower lips can be supported with thicker fillers. Perlane®, more viscous than Restylane®, is great for this purpose, but it is not yet available in the United States. We use Restylane® for the lip border and corners and use Sculptra® in the marionette line area to support the corners of the mouth.

When loss of skin tone and resilience are apparent, results can be further enhanced with skin tightening and collagen stimulating procedures using Thermage®, non-ablative lasers, and intense pulsed light. Minute vertical wrinkles in the upper lip vermilion border can be eradicated with Restylane® or Cosmoplast®, used together to augment the upper lip border. The Cosmoplast® has an anesthetic agent mixed with it. Injecting it first in the lip border will numb the lip and can make the remaining treatment with Restylane® or Perlane® easier.

Deeper, longer vertical upper lip furrows can be filled with Restylane® or Captique™, after being relaxed with Botox® across the upper lip border. Combining Botox® and filling can provide effective resolution of upper lip vertical wrinkles and furrows without downtime.

What do we do if there are many fine wrinkles and deep furrows, and there is significant upper lip skin sun damage?

This is when laser resurfacing is worthwhile. The lip orbicularis oris is relaxed with Botox®. Then the upper lip is resurfaced with the carbon dioxide or erbium:YAG laser. This provides the most effective long-term results but requires about four to five days of healing with the erbium laser and one week with the carbon dioxide laser. The length of time that the lip will remain pink depends on the laser we use, the power setting, and the number of times we pass the laser over the tissue. After the healing has begun, the upper lip can be camouflaged with makeup that serves as a physical sun block and protects the new skin, allowing it to heal more quickly.

We have an increasing palette of fillers to choose from as we sculpt, adjust, and reinflate facial structures and lip contours.

The depressor anguli oris is the muscle that pulls down the corners of the mouth. It can be treated with Botox® to slightly raise the corners of the mouth, making Restylane®, Perlane®, Sculptra®, or Radiesse™ more effective when filling marionette lines. These fillers can be layered to create a complete effect. Sculptra® can fill in larger, broader areas; Sculptra® or Radiesse™ can accentuate or establish bony contours; deeper remaining linear irregularities can be filled with Perlane® or Radiesse™; and fine lines filled with Restylane®.

CHAPTER 14

Non-Surgical Neck Rejuvenation

The neck plays an important role in how we are perceived. Neck characteristics and qualities are idealized in the perception of feminine beauty and youth in different cultures. It is widely accepted that a long, thin, slender swanlike neck is a pleasing and feminine characteristic of a woman's appearance. A different set of characteristics is assigned to the male neck. The ideal man's neck is described as strong, muscular, or thick, giving an aggressive and dominant quality. Redundant folds, sagging skin, superfluous fatty tissue, double chins, and wrinkles do not fit into any ideal of neck beauty.

Neck rejuvenation has a balancing and complementary role in the whole approach to a youthful appearance. The chin and jawline frame the facial characteristics. The quality and texture of the skin, the amount and firmness of the fat, the strength of the muscles, thickness and form, anatomy and prominence of the glands, thyroid cartilage and the surrounding bones are all key elements that influence the appearance of the neck. The bony structures of the face, neck, and upper chest provide the framework for the attachment of the soft tissues.

The inevitable changes of time upon the tissues can affect the neck to different degrees. The skin loses its resiliency and becomes wrinkled and saggy. The platysma muscle may atrophy, becoming thin and forming platysmal bands which become noticeable, running from the chin down to the collar bone. Submental fat increases and results in a double chin. Jowls become more prominent and begin to sag, further altering the midfacial contours by dragging down facial tissues. These multifactorial changes cannot be corrected with any single non-invasive treatment. Until now, the choices available for neck rejuvenation have been largely surgical.

SURGICAL NECK REJUVENATION TECHNIQUES
Cervicofacial rhytidectomy
Submandibular gland resection
Facialplasty
Contour threads lift
Deep plane facelift
Suture suspension neck lift
Platysmaplasty
S-Lift with O and M sutures

The goal of surgical intervention is to restore youthful facial anatomy by removing redundant tissue, repositioning lax tissue, physically tightening the underlying muscles, and supporting tissue.

We have developed an innovative non-invasive, non-surgical four step approach to neck rejuvenation. The goal of these therapies is to rejuvenate the neck by promoting collagen remodeling and regeneration rather than by aggressive surgical intervention and removal of neck tissue.

4 STAGES OF NON-SURGICAL NECK REJUVENATION	
STEP ONE	Botulinum toxin injections to relax platysmal banding, reduce the downward pull of the platysma, reduce neck wrinkling
STEP TWO	Thermage® to tighten neck skin; stacked Thermage® applications to reduce localized submental (double chin) fat accumulation

STEP THREE	Phosphatidylcholine injections to reduce residual localized fat accumulation
STEP FOUR	Skin texture and resilience are corrected with CO2Cellulair™, Restylane Vital, superficial chemical peels, cosmeceutical skincare, non-ablative lasers, and IPL (Intense Pulsed Light) to further enhance the Thermage® effect

Minimally invasive neck rejuvenation can be achieved with a combination of multiple treatments and techniques with different mechanisms of action. The ultimate goal is to combine these actions in order to get the maximum neck rejuvenating effect with minimum healing and recovery time.

Surgical techniques of neck rejuvenation may target specific types of tissues (skin, fat, muscle) depending on their contribution to the aging effect on the neck. Unlike the non-invasive approach, the healing time and recovery period after surgical procedures ranges from several weeks to several months. The bruising and swelling that follows surgical procedures may restrict your lifestyle and activities. For this reason many of our patients prefer less invasive therapies, even if they may to need repeat treatments to maintain the desirable effect. Even the menu of non-surgical options gives you the choice between a series of smaller procedures with no downtime, and a slightly stronger procedure that involves several days of downtime. Your work, social schedule, and tolerance for downtime are paramount in selecting a treatment plan that meets your needs.

What are your priorities?

Sitting directly in front of you, we will examine you at rest and in animation. We will hand you a mirror and ask you to point to the areas that bother you. This gives us an opportunity to establish your priorities, to discuss all the options, and to set realistic expectations about what we can and cannot achieve.

We examine you at rest and while you are speaking, from the front and from each side. We will ask you to raise your chin and then to depress your chin to your chest. The quality, texture, pigmentation, and resilience of your neck skin are important considerations. We note the amount and location of fatty deposits, the prominence of the glands under your jaw, and the extent and location of neck muscle bands. Our observations are correlated to your list of complaints, concerns, and priorities.

Post-Treatment Course

We explain what to expect after each treatment session, when you can expect to notice improvement, if you will be bruised and swollen, and for how long. These are the questions that you will want answered. We will also review the type and frequency of the different options that you will need for maintenance to sustain the effects and benefits of these treatments.

Treatment Options

We will recommend a customized treatment plan based on what we see and on what you would like to have improved. Just because the aging changes you see may seem to be similar to your girlfriend, does not necessarily mean that our proposed treatment plan will be the same. The appearance of each patient's neck may be the result of different causes. For example, consider the development of a double chin. The cause may be excess fat, redundant skin, or a hypertrophic muscle. It may all look the same to you, but each cause requires a different method of correction.

Our personal approach to rejuvenation of the neck using non-invasive techniques is based on a very simple concept: use multiple tissue specific treatments and combine the effects of those treatments to achieve the best result. The rationale behind this thinking is that the effect of each tissue on the appearance of the neck has a different underlying mechanism. Skin wrinkles because of tissue change caused by sun damage and aging tissue; the platysma muscle weakens, separates, and forms bands; and submental fat accumulates.

CATEGORIES OF NON-INVASIVE NECK TREATMENTS

• Relax the neck musculature

• Tighten the skin

• Reduce the amount of excess fat

• Improve the texture, tone, and resilience of the skin

Our personal experience has shown us that performing some treatments first helps improve the effectiveness of other subsequent treatments. Relaxing the neck musculature and reducing unwanted fat from the submental area can provide an improved anatomical foundation for the subsequent aesthetic improvement of the overlying skin and yield the desired neck contour. We recommend addressing issues of skin quality and texture as a final step after performing skin-tightening and recontouring treatments. However, to speed up the process we often begin skin texture treatments while we are awaiting the final effects of skin tightening procedures

STEP ONE: RELAXING THE MUSCLES

Relaxing the muscles of the neck using botulinum toxin can improve the appearance of the neck and prepare the overlying tissues for maximum rejuvenation with complementary treatments. We routinely use botulinum toxin before skin tightening procedures. The effect of relaxing the muscles and reducing the muscle bands and the overlying skin wrinkles of the neck also provides a smoother scaffold for the new skin collagen that will be stimulated with non-ablative lasers, intense pulse light or Thermage®. Botox® not only affects the injected muscles but also extends to all the soft tissues connected to these muscles. We suspect that Botox® itself in some way stimulates collagen regeneration.

The platysma muscle is actually a pair of thin muscles originating from the deep tissue and skin of the lower neck and upper chest, extending laterally toward the shoulder and back, and upward to the angle of the jaw and the skin below to the mouth. Its main functions are drawing the corners of the mouth downward and assisting in opening of the mouth by depressing the jawbone. Loss of muscle tone due to aging may result in a separation of the one smooth flat muscle into two vertical muscle bands in the neck. Loss of elasticity of the neck skin that covers these muscles will also form a necklace of horizontal wrinkles.

Our use of a specially compounded topical anesthetic cream and ice compresses applied over the neck muscle band will make this treatment virtually painless. Although we try very hard to avoid it, there is always the possibility of getting a bruise. While we grasp the skin and the platysmal band between our fingers, we give a series of very tiny injections just under the skin band along the length of the band. We use just enough Botox® to relax and smooth the neck cords but not enough to cause the very rare complication of swallowing difficulty.

Besides relaxing playsmal bands Botox® may be used to reduce horizontal necklace wrinkles as well. The relaxing effect of Botox® will begin to appear three to five days after the injection. Because it may take up to ten days for the full effect to take place, we routinely schedule a follow-up visit for one to two weeks following the initial injection.

Botox® may also be used to improve the appearance of jowls and elevate the corners of the mouth by reducing the action of the platysma and the muscle that pulls down the corner of the mouth (depressor anguli oris muscle). Maintenance treatments every three to four months will maintain the Botox® effect and enhance the longevity of the other non-ablative procedures like laser skin rejuvenation and Thermage®.

STEP TWO: SKIN TIGHTENING

Tightening the skin and sculpting the fat under the chin is the next step in non-invasive neck rejuvenation. The more effectively the muscles underlying the skin have been relaxed, the more effective radiofrequency skin tightening will be. Until recently, we only had surgical techniques such as neck lift and platysma plasty to offer. Laser resurfacing of the neck skin has not been particularly useful since healing of the neck skin takes a long time and is unpredictable. Thermage® causes collagen shrinkage and new collagen deposition followed by long-term collagen remodeling.

Pretreatment of the neck muscles with botulinum toxin is ideally done one week before to facilitate the lifting and tightening of the treatment by reducing resistance. Since many of our patients come from great distances, we may do Botox® on the same day as Thermage®. Most of the collagen remodeling stimulated by the radio frequency treatment takes place during the first three to four months although the final result may not be visible for four to six months. This is how long Botox® lasts, so they work in perfect combination. The collagen in the skin is tightening and lifting while the Botox® is relaxing the muscles that would have been wrinkling and pulling down the skin.

When we first started performing this procedure we applied a temporary stencil grid to the skin in the areas to be treated to ensure that we were treating all areas equally and not overlapping. Now we apply the treatment in what we call "vectors" imaginary lines that we want to tighten. We go over the areas to tighten the skin in a way to support the areas that sag the most; the submental area (under the chin) and the lateral (outside) aspects of the neck as far back as the strap muscles. We do not treat the front of the neck over the trachea or esophagus. To make our vectors more accurate and to treat the areas that sag the most of the neck, we will have you sitting comfortably in the upright position, facing away from the side being treated, with your chin elevated.

CO2Cellulair™ and the Alma ST handpiece enhance the skin tightening and skin texture effects of Thermage. They are repeated on a weekly basis for four to five weeks beginning one month after the Thermage treatment. They are virtually painless and without downtime.

Pain Management for Special Areas

Where there is extra fat and skin under the chin, we treat the area many times (even up to ten or twenty times). We call it "pulse stacking" and use it in areas where we want to melt subcutaneous fat. The power that we use will be determined by you. We want you to feel the heat of each treatment, but we do not want it to be painful. We will give you a discomfort rating scale of "0 to 4." You will rate the treatment as a "0" if you feel nothing. You will rate the treatment as a "4" if it is intolerably hot. We want each treatment to feel like a "2".

If the treatment feels more than a "2," we lower the power. We pass over the area five to six times, then lower the power one notch, then pass over the areas another five to six times. We continue lowering the power and passing over the area until we have treated the area under the chin with at least 100 pulses.

In the other areas of the neck where the skin is thinner and there is little or no fat, we will use lower power settings and grasp the loose skin between our finger when treating it. For sagging jowls, we will treat above and below the jawline and extending two finger widths below the jawline.

By the end of the treatment, a subtle tightening and lifting is evident. We usually treat one side at a time so that you can look in the mirror and compare the treated and untreated sides.

Most patients only require one treatment. After three to four months, you can have a second treatment if you would like even further improvement. In addition to the tightening effect, there is usually some improvement in the overall skin quality. This could be explained by the formation and deposition of new collagen. The longevity of the effect may be several years, and repeat treatments may be necessary to maintain or enhance the result.

STEP THREE: CONTOURING FAT

Subcutaneous submental fat may give the appearance of a double chin, blunt the jaw line (cervicomental angle), and cause sagging of the neck skin. Fat in this location, under the skin, is responsive to non-invasive techniques. Remaining submental fat after Thermage® can be treated with fat melting injections or liposuction. Subplatysmal fat lies deeper, under the muscle, and is not accessible without surgery.

FAT DISSOLVING TECHNIQUES

Phosphatidylcholine is an enzyme that dissolves fat. It is useful for improving neck contours and for diminishing any fatty tissue under the chin in the submental area which may remain after Thermage® treatments. It has been used for many years in Brazil, Germany, and Italy as a lipid lowering drug (Lipostabil® (Aventis)). The medication Lipostabil® (Aventis) has also been used off label as an injectable fat dissolving agent in Europe and South America. It is not approved by the FDA in the United States, but the enzyme phosphatidyl choline is available through compounding pharmacies. Five to ten small injections are given during each session. These are followed by mild itching and swelling that may last several weeks. In some cases, it may take ten to fourteen days to notice a visible improvement. Usually two to five treatments spaced about three to four weeks apart are effective.

Although injections of phosphatidyl choline have been reportedly successful in treating prominent periorbital fat—lower lid bags—we do not use it around the eye and orbital area because its effect is not controllable and there are too many delicate structures around the eyes. We have also found that it is not practical to use on the face to reduce cheek fat pockets and jowls because there is usually a significant amount of swelling following these injections that may last several weeks.

Mesotherapy is a category of treatments that involve the injection of different substances within the skin. Since many of the other substances injected in meso-therapy protocols do not have well documented clinical indications or effects, and we do not use them.

Submental Liposuction

We can also remove any residual fatty deposits of the neck and jowls by using tiny incisions and tumescent liposuction performed under local anesthesia with intravenous sedation. With the tumescent technique we use a large amount of local anesthesia to make the procedure virtually painless and with minimal or no bleeding at all. This makes the procedure safer with minimal healing time. First, we mark the areas of fat deposits to be removed with you sitting in the upright position. Tiny incisions are hidden in the crease underneath your chin and under your earlobes so that a thin metal tube called a cannula can be placed under the skin and used to suck out the fat. In some cases, we will use intravenous sedation if you prefer to be sleepy during surgery. The key advantage of this technique is rapid recovery. After the procedure, an elastic band is worn under your chin for three to five days to reduce swelling. You can usually return to work and to normal activities over a long weekend.

STEP FOUR: REJUVENATION OF SKIN TEXTURE AND PIGMENT

Photodamage plays a significant role in the degeneration of neck skin. Years of UV exposure contribute to the development of wrinkles, poikiloderma (red veins and blotches), and actinic keratoses (raised, flat pigments and scaly sunspots). The treatment of post-menopausal hair growth on the chin and submental areas must also be considered. The goal is to improve the texture, tone, and resilience of the skin, which can be accomplished with several treatment modalities.

Superficial peels are the least invasive of all skin treatments for the neck. They essentially exfoliate the top layers of the epidermis and result in an improvement in overall skin texture. We recommend initially a series of at least five peels, one per week, to accelerate early improvement and accentuate the effects of skincare. We typically start with a 70 percent buffered solution and advance to higher concentrations during subsequent treatments. We conclude the treatment by applying a moisturizing Crystal C gel and sun block. We apply B+Z Lipocel cream to the neck for added moisturization. To maintain and prolong the effects of these treatments, we recommend the daily use of sunscreen, which is essential to prevent further sun damage. If you will not use sunscreen on a daily basis (and this means every day rain or shine), continued skincare is pointless.

For treating more advanced sun damage there are several options. Photorejuvenation of the skin with non-ablative light emitting devices offers impressive results with minimal downtime and discomfort. Intense pulsed light devices (IPL) can be used to treat brown and red lesions of the neck skin including blotchy skin (poikiloderma) and broken capillaries. Photodynamic therapy (PDT), using Levulan™ and a blue light source or IPL, will require four to five days downtime (extreme redness) but each treatment is equivalent to three IPL sessions. And light TCA peels can be very helpful to reduce mottled pigmentation. We are also on the threshold of the development of two new lasers whose effects are midway between ablative and non-ablative therapies—Fraxel™ and Plasma lasers. Since ablative laser treatment of the neck is unpredictable and healing time can be lengthy, these new lasers may be helpful in the future.

IPL, PDT, TCA and semi-ablative lasers (Fraxel™ and Plasma) can also be used to soften the demarcation between a laser-resurfaced face and a sun-damaged neck. Collagen regeneration and wrinkle ablation will also benefit from this approach. Four or five treatment sessions of IPL or Fraxel™ may be necessary to achieve the desired effect, while one session of TCA or Plasma laser may do the job. PDT may require one or two treatment sessions.

Before treating darker skinned patients with any IPL treatment, we apply a test patch to the skin behind the ear. We observe the area for one half hour and then reexamine the area again in one week. If we do not see any redness and there is no hyperpigmentation by the next week, we can proceed with the treatment. If you have a tan, we cannot do any resurfacing treatment because this will increase your chances of hyperpigmentation. Hyperpigmentation is most likely temporary, but may last several months. You will need frequent glycolic acid peels and have to use our Clarifying Lotion at bedtime.

We begin the IPL treatment by applying a clear chilled gel to the skin of your neck. The IPL crystal is then placed on top of the gel and we cover your eyes with goggles. You may have a warm tingling sensation while the procedure is being performed. We can also apply numbing cream to your face before the treatment, if desired. We begin with low power settings, and raise the power slightly with each subsequent treatment, until we get the desired result without making your face too red.

The dynamically cooled long pulse 1320nm Nd:YAG (Cool touch™ II, Cutera, Brisbane, CA) is a non-ablative laser on the menu of treatments for aging and photodamaged skin. It can improve the appearance of wrinkles, reduce pore size, and improve skin texture. We recommend four to six monthly treatments. The results improve gradually over three to six months. This laser as well as the 1064nm (Cool Glide) laser can be used on all skin types. Their main action is stimulation of fibroblasts to form new collagen in the skin. The epidermal layer of the skin is cooled while the beam heats the deep tissues to protect the surface of the skin. At the conclusion of the treatment, mild redness is treated with cool compresses. In our practices we have replaced Cool Touch treatments with a combination of CO2Cellulair™ and Alma ST treatments. There is less discomfort and these treatments are more cost effective.

For long-term hair removal, many laser devices are available—Alexandrite, Diode, and Nd:YAG (neodymium: yttrium-aluminum-garnet). For the hair follicle to absorb the maximum laser energy effectively and to avoid singeing of long hairs, we shave the area and apply topical anesthetic cream for 20 minutes. Chilled clear aloe gel applied to the area serves as a coupling gel to minimize the scattering of light and as a cooling and soothing medium to maximize your comfort. The brass-cooling tip of the Cool Glide laser cools the skin immediately before and after treatment. Because not all hairs are at the anagen growth phase at the time of treatment, it usually takes four to six treatment sessions spaced three to four weeks apart for best results.

Afterword

Lately it seems that virtually every doctor is offering Botox®, laser photofacials, or some other aesthetic treatment. The myriad of choices facing the average person is both overwhelming and incomprehensible. Although there are many competent physicians out there, in many cases these kinds of services are being offered by doctors with inadequate knowledge of the intricate workings of the muscles of the face or the eyes and their delicate and fragile interplay. Finally two brilliant eyelid surgeons with decades of experience, who have been on the cutting edge in both Brazil and New York, are sharing their experience with the lay person. Previously their many books and papers were strictly for other doctors. Much of their practices had been devoted to people with extreme disfigurement following accidents or tumor surgery and others in need of corrective eyelid surgery. Their practice has evolved and embraced the most innovative techniques and equipment in the world to truly beautifeye the average person. This is a book that anyone considering a surgical or noninvasive procedure can not afford to miss. For less than one tenth the cost of a consultation, this book can save you from spending thousands of dollars on an unnecessary facelift.

—*John Aslanian*
Oz Garcia's Longevity Lounge
New York, NY

Resources

www.eye-lift.com
www.beautifeye.com
www.asoprs.org

Glossary

A

Actinic keratoses—(Solar keratosis) a lesion that is dry, scaly, rough, and tan or pink caused by sun exposure; considered precancerous

Alpha hydroxy acids (AHA's)—a group of naturally occurring substances derived from sugar cane, apples, and citrus fruit that are used in various concentrations to exfoliate the superficial layers of skin

Aponeurosis—any of the broad flat sheets of dense fibrous collagenous connective tissue that cover, invest, and form the terminations and attachments of various muscles.

Arnica montana—a homeopathic remedy that reduces bruising and swelling

B

Basal cell carcinoma—the most common form of skin cancer of one of the innermost cells of the deeper epidermis of the skin

Blepharitis—an inflammation of the eyelid that may occur at the margins of the eyelids when the oil glands become irritated

Blepharoplasty—surgery to repair a defect or correct the eyelid to improve both form and function of the eyelid; cosmetic eyelid surgery

Blepharospasm—spasmodic winking and closure from involuntary contraction of the orbicularis oculi muscle of the eyelids

Blepharoptosis—drooping or abnormal relaxation of the upper eyelid, can be congenital or acquired; can block peripheral vision

Brow depressor muscles—the muscles which pull down the eyebrows—the corrugator, depressor superciliaris, the orbicularis oculi muscles

Brow lift—helps eliminate horizontal lines in the forehead, corrects ptosis of the eyebrows, and relieves upper lid hooding

C

Canthus—either the inner or the outer angles formed by the meeting of the upper and lower eyelids. The outer—or lateral—canthus should make a more acute angle

Carbon dioxide laser—Carbon dioxide laser resurfacing creates partial thickness vaporization of the most superficial layer of cells that cover the skin (epidermis). The next deepest layer of skin creates a new surface and forms new collagen in the underlying dermis. The carbon dioxide laser can also be used as a highly effective surgical instrument

Conjunctiva—The transparent membrane that covers the sclera toward the front of the eye and that also lines the inside of the eyelids.

Cornea—The transparent, curved structure on the front of the eye that focuses incoming light rays—the "watch crystal" of the eye. This is the tissue treated during refractive (Lasik) surgery

Corrugator muscles—muscles just above the brow and between the brows that create frown lines

D

Dermatochalasis—redundant and lax, upper eyelid skin and muscle

Dermis—the deep layer of the skin

Diode laser—used for laser hair removal, the safest of the layers used for long-lasting hair removal; it can be used on darkly pigmented patients

Diplopia—a disorder of vision in which two images of a single object are seen because of unequal action of the eye muscles—also called double vision

Dry eye syndrome—a drying out of the surface of the cornea caused by a lack of tears or by a chemical imbalance in the tears; its symptoms include a foreign body sensation, burning, and photophobia; there can also be a reaction of too much tearing

E

Ectropion—a turning out of the eyelid; can result in a malposition of the tear drain

Edema—an abnormal infiltration and excess accumulation of serous fluid in connective tissue following trauma or surgery

Endoscopic—a method of examining through a small opening using an endoscope, a narrow, flexible fiber optic instrument that conducts light.

Endoscopic brow lift—the elevation of the eyebrows using an endoscope through small scale incisions

Entropion—a turning in of the eyelids that may cause the eyelashes to abrade the cornea.

Epidermis—outer layer of cells that line the superficial skin

Erbium: YAG—a laser that provides tissue ablation without secondary thermal effects; requires less healing time than carbon dioxide laser resurfacing

Erythema—redness of the skin following surgery, laser applications, or laser resurfacing

F

Flashlamp—a lamp for producing a brief but intense flash of light used especially to deliver light that is absorbed by different colored skin lesions (red or brown)

Frontalis muscle—muscle of the entire forehead, elevates eyebrow and creates horizontal furrows

G

Glabella—the smooth prominence between the eyebrows that becomes furrowed when the corrugator (frowning) muscles are overactive

H

Hematoma—a mass of clotted blood that forms as a result of trauma, surgery, or laser application

Hyaluronic Acid—a natural compound found in every organ of the body and in every living species

Hydrophilic—having a strong affinity for water; dissolving readily in water

Hydroquinone—a powerful skin bleaching agent

Hyperpigmentation—too much pigmentation; dark areas of skin; may be caused by inflammation

Hypopigmentation—less than normal pigment; light skin; may follow inflammation

I

Inferior scleral show—a malposition of the lower lid— lower lid retraction—exposing the inferior aspect of the eye; may result in corneal drying and increased tearing

Intense pulsed light (IPL)—a well-recognized treatment option for improving the appearance of photoaging, including the appearance of redness, veins, rough texture, fine wrinkles, and mottled pigmentation; uses a flash lamp to deliver light, filtering out different wave lengths

K

Kojic acid—used with retinoids and hydroquinone to reduce hyperpigmentation

L

Lacrimal duct (nasolacrimal duct)—tear drainage duct; passageway through the bone of the nose that carries the tears from the lacrimal sac to the interior of the nose

Lateral canthoplasty—tightening and repositioning of the lateral canthal tendon that supports the lower lid

Lateral canthus—outer corner of the eye, supported by the lateral canthal tendon; laxity of this tendon can cause rounding of the lateral canthal angle

Lateral hooding—excess fold of skin between the eyebrow and the outer portion of the upper eyelid can interfere with the peripheral visual fields

Levator muscle—this muscle is the primary muscle used in opening the upper lid. The levator muscle starts back above the eyeball, courses over the top, descends into the eyelid, and attaches to the tarsus, above the eyelid margin. Its function is to lift the eyelid out of the line of vision

M

Melasma—a skin hyperpigmentation condition presenting as brown patches on the face. Both sides of the face are usually affected. The most common sites are the cheeks, bridge of nose, forehead, and upper lip.

Micropigmentation—semi-permanent makeup applied with a delicate tattooing

Milia—a small pearly firm non-inflammatory elevation of the skin (as of the face) due to retention of keratin in an oil gland duct blocked by a thin layer of epithelium

N

Nasal jugal groove—groove between side of nose and cheek

Nasolabial fold—fold from corner of nostril to outer corner of mouth

Non-ablative lasers—lasers that can be used with little or no downtime non-ablative laser devices classically emit energy in coherent wavelengths within the near infrared to infrared spectrum

O

Orbicularis oculi—muscle that closes the eye; directly beneath the skin; circles around the upper and lower eyelids

Orbit—the boney cavity in the skull where the eyeballs, eye muscles, nerves and blood vessels are protected. Orbital fat within this cavity protects these delicate structures. When this fat is displaced forward, it becomes visible as a lower lid bag

Orbital Rim—edge of the boney orbit; helps protect eyes from injury

P

Photothermolysis—created by a filtered flashlamp non-coherent intense pulsed light source (IPL). It is used to treat small blood vessels and to ablate broken capillaries on the nose and cheeks

Pigment—the chemical compound in cells that creates the color of a tissue

Platysma—a pair of muscles originating from the lower neck and upper chest, extending laterally to the anterior surface of the deltoid muscles and inserting at the inferior border of the mandible and the skin inferior to the mouth.

Platysmal bands—vertical neck bands that form where there is laxity of the platysma muscle

PolyLactic acid—Sculptra®, a synthetic non-immunogenic, absorbable substance that is mixed with sterile water and anesthetic that is effective in filling out depressed facial areas or areas of muscle atrophy.

Prolapsing orbital fat—lower lid bags caused by orbital fat that moves forward

Procerus muscle—one of the muscles that bring the brow down. This muscle arises from radix (base) of the nose and inserts into the forehead; can create the horizontal furrow across the bridge of the nose

Ptosis (toe-sis)—drooping particularly of eyelids and brows. Eyelid ptosis—blepharotosis—may block the field of vision. Brow ptosis causes redundancy of the upper lid fold

Purpura—characterized by patches of purplish discoloration resulting from blood into the skin and mucous membranes. Can be caused by dye lasers

R

Radio frequency—any of the electromagnetic wave frequencies that lie in a range extending from below 3 kilohertz to about 300 gigahertz. This energy is used to heat the deeper layers of the skin—Thermage®

Retinoid—topical peeling agent that reduces actinic (sun-related) skin changes

Retrobulbar hematoma—bleeding behind the eye caused by surgery or trauma

Rosacea—a vascular condition characterized by reddish bumps and blood vessels on the central areas of the face

S

Sclera—the white outer coat of the eyeball

Silicone—a liquid injectable permanent filling agent that has been used since the 1940's

Solar lentigenes—dark brown spots that occur on sun-exposed areas of skin

Stratum corneum—outermost layer of skin or epidermis known as the horny layer.

Subcutaneous—under the skin

Subdermal—under the dermis

T

Tear duct—the canaliculus—a short canal leading from a minute orifice on a small elevation at the medial angle of each eyelid (the punctum) to the lacrimal sac

Tear trough deformity—depression along the medial aspect of the lower lid adjacent to the medial orbital bone; can create a shadow

Trans-blepharoplasty internal brow suspension—a brow lift performed through a blepharoplasty incision

Transconjunctival—through the inner lining of the eyelid

Transconjunctival blepharoplasty—a lower eyelift performed through the inside of the lower lid without a skin incision

Trichloracetic acid (TCA)—TCA is the most common agent for medium depth peels. It is used in different concentrations for peels of varying depths

Index

BOSNIAK + ZILKHA

EYELID AND FACIAL PRODUCTS

B+Z Beautif-Eye™ Cream   .5 oz $195.00

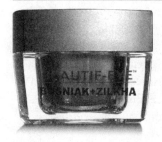

This revolutionary product is the first eyelid skin product created by eyelid surgeons. It has a proprietary blend of unique brazilian rain forest antioxidants and moisturizers. Its first visible effects begin less than one half hour after applying it - lightening dark circles, softening fine lines, and decreasing puffiness. Continued use every morning and evening will increase its therapeutic action.

B+Z Non-Alcohol Toner

A soothing facial toner, make-up remover   8 oz $45.00
and lash cleanser

B+Z Gentle Cleanser

A mild, non-irritating, non-drying cleanser   8 oz $45.00

B+Z AHA Cleanser

Excellent for acne control and can be used   7 oz $45.00
as a shaving gel

B+Z Smoothing Lotion (AHA face/body lotion)

Effective for acne control   8 oz $45.00

B+Z Retinoic Acid 0.05% Hydroquinone Lotion Rx

Prescription strength lotion for pigment contol   1.5 oz $110.00
Only available for sale to our patients

B+Z Retinoic Acid 0.07% Hydroquinone Lotion Rx

Prescription strength lotion for pigment contol   1.5 oz $110.00
Only available for sale to our patients

B+Z Retinoic Acid Hydroquinone Hand & Foot Cream Rx

Prescription strength lotion for pigment contol   30 gm $110.00
Only available for sale to our patients

B+Z Crystal C Serum

Superb moisturizing anti-oxidant serum   1 oz $90.00

B+Z Satin Serum

Revitalizes skin's protective lipid layer   .5 oz $95.00

B+Z Lipicel Cream Moist

A richly nourishing rehydrating cream   2 oz $75.00

B+Z Acne Prone AHA Smoothing Gel

Potent acne control   4 oz $55.00

Notes